Continuing Care Retirement Communities

Political, Social, and Financial Issues

Continuing Care Retirement Communities

Political, Social, and Financial Issues

Ian A. Morrison, Ruth Bennett,
Susana Frisch and Barry J. Gurland
Editors

The Haworth Press
New York • London

Continuing Care Retirement Communities: Political, Social, and Financial Issues has also been published as *Journal of Housing for the Elderly,* Volume 3, Numbers 1/2, Spring/Summer 1985.

The Haworth Press, Inc., 28 East 22 Street, New York, NY 10010-6194
EUROSPAN/Haworth, 3 Henrietta Street, London WC2E 8LU England

Library of Congress Cataloging-In-Publication Data
Main entry under title:

Continuing care retirement communities.

"Also published as Journal of housing for the elderly, volume 3, numbers 1-2, spring-summer, 1985"—T.p. verso.
    Based on proceedings of a conference held June 9-10, 1983 at the Kellogg Conf. Center, Columbia University and organized by the Center for Geriatrics and Gerontology, Columbia University Faculty of Medicine and New York State Office of Mental Health.
    Includes bibliographies.
    1. Life care communities—United States—Congresses. 2. Life care communities—United States—Finance—Congresses. 3. Life care communities—Law and legislation—United States—Congresses. 4. Life care communities—New York (State)—Case Studies—Congresses. 5. Life care communities—Pennsylvania—Case studies—Congresses. I. Morrison, Ian A. II. Center for Geriatrics and Gerontology (New York, N.Y.) III. New York (State). Office of Mental Health.
HV1454.2.U6C65   1986   362.1'6'0973   85-8669
ISBN 0-86656-384-9

Continuing Care Retirement Communities: Political, Social, and Financial Issues

Journal of Housing for the Elderly
Volume 3, Numbers 1/2

CONTENTS

PART II: LEGAL, FINANCIAL AND ETHICAL ISSUES

PART III: EVOLVING MANAGEMENT
STRUCTURES: A CASE STUDY

Preface

This volume is an outgrowth of a conference sponsored by Columbia University's Center for Geriatrics and Gerontology on the topic of Continuing Care Retirement Communities in New York State: Past, Present and Future, held June 9-10, 1983 at Columbia University. The need for this conference was first made apparent to us by a meeting with Dr. Ian Morrison, President of Greer-Woodycrest Foundation who was then considering the feasibility of developing a continuing care retirement community in New York State. The continuing care retirement community is one distinct option that the elderly might wish to evaluate in relation to their diverse needs and resources.

As people age they become more diverse; their inherited constitution, early upbringing and adult experiences interact in a rich variety of combinations and permutations producing a unique evolution of their thinking, behavior and needs. Adding to this diversity is the reaction to the development of age-related physical, mental or social problems, offset by maturing assets and achievements. The diverse needs of elderly people require consideration of diverse solutions.

It is apparent that the continuing care retirement community is regarded as a viable option for serving their needs by at least some elderly people in many parts of this country. However, this arrangement while being encouraged in some regions has been discouraged in others. We can usefully explore this discrepancy and lay out the issues so that they can be discussed among protagonists and antagonists of all viewpoints.

The staff members of the Center for Geriatrics and Gerontology who hosted the conference that led to this volume are naturally inclined to hold strong views about many issues related to aging, but in this instance we have chosen to remain neutral because we want to include proponents of a wide range of possible conflicting views.

The contributors to this volume were participants in the conference and are major developers of the thinking and practice in this field dealing with options for living arrangements for the elderly. The work of the conference was effected through a series of speakers and also workshops which were of equal importance. Questions raised after each speaker were devoted to clarification of issues to be later discussed in detail in the workshops and reported in the concluding session. Many of the speakers took part in the workshops to give the audience a chance to make a more searching exploration of their views.

It is our hope that the detailed discussion of these issues contained in this volume might give rise to fresh perspectives and modes of action.

Barry Gurland
Director, Center for Geriatrics and Gerontology
Columbia University

Acknowledgements

This volume is based on the proceedings of the conference on Continuing Care Retirement Communities in New York State: Past, Present and Future, held June 9-10, 1983 at the Kellogg Conference Center, Columbia University of the City of New York. The Conference was organized by the Center for Geriatrics and Gerontology, Columbia University Faculty of Medicine and New York State Office of Mental Health.

Thanks and appreciation are offered to the many people who generously contributed time and effort to plan and develop the conference as well as edit this volume. The following persons are recognized for their participation:

Conference Planning Group

Ruth Bennett
Deputy Director
Center for Geriatrics and
   Gerontology

Barry J. Gurland
Director
Center for Geriatrics and
   Gerontology

Ian Morrison
President
Greer-Woodycrest
Children's Services

Lloyd Nurick
Director
New York Association of
   Homes and Services
   for the Aging

Corinne Plummer
Deputy Commissioner
Division of Adult Services
N.Y.S. Department of Social
   Services

Paul A. Wagner
President
NPO/TASK FORCE, Inc.

George M. Warner
Special Health Care Advisor
Office of Health Systems
   Management
N.Y.S. Department of Health

David E. Wilder
Deputy Director
Center for Geriatrics and
   Gerontology

Conference Sponsors

The Conference was supported by generous contributions from the following organizations:

The Dyson-Kissner-Moran Corporation
James A. Eddy Memorial Foundation
Greer-Woodycrest Children's Services
The Hoffman Partnership, Inc.
Laventhol & Horwath
Loeb & Troper
Merrill Lynch White Weld
Peat, Marwick, Mitchell & Co.
Herbert J. Sims & Co., Inc.

Editorial Committee

Ruth Bennett   Ian Morrison
Susana Frisch   Paul Wagner
Barry Gurland   George Warner

Conference Staff

Special thanks are extended to Mrs. Susana Frisch for her valuable assistance in coordinating the activities related to all aspects of the conference.

We also wish to thank all those who served as conference staff and who efficiently got everything and everyone to the right place at the right time.

Last but not least special recognition is due to Ms. Deborah Israel who patiently typed several versions of the manuscripts which make up this volume.

Prologue and Introduction

Ian A. Morrison

Three or four years ago when the organization, of which I am president, decided that massive changes in public social welfare policy in the state of New York mandated that we look at alternatives to some of the things we were doing, I was led into a field in which I was totally innocent, and absolutely ignorant. That was the field of the elderly and the concept of a "life-care community." My early years at Columbia University paid off as I began the long trek to find out what was going on in the United States and what was happening in New York State in regard to life-care communities for the elderly. It took me about ten minutes to discover that there was nothing going on in New York State. I did not know Lloyd Nurick in those days, nor the great things he had accomplished. (See Chapter 9 of this volume.)

The reality was that in New York State there was an absolute dearth of information on the subject. So we began the search in Washington to learn what many of you have known for years about this field. We knew, from our own information in this state, that there was a pent-up desire on the part of people who were approaching 60, 65 and 70 for the kind of facilities that they had seen in New Jersey, Pennsylvania, and Florida as well as in other places but could not find in New York. Enough people of that type had talked to us to indicate that with the assets and the resources—the land, the board and the staff that we had at Woodycrest—it was an area in which we ought to be able to accomplish something.

As we began the study, which was essentially a feasibility study, we ran into interesting people and, fortunately for me, one of the first that I ran into was Frank Elliot (see Chapter 6) of the Life Care Society of America, Inc. in Pennsylvania. He cut through a lot of red tape, a lot of myths and a lot of "do-goodism" as he talked to me about the realities of creating and running a proprietary organi-

---

Ian A. Morrison is President of Greer-Woodycrest, Millbrook, N.Y.

zation of this type. Later on we met with Monsignor Fahey, whose perspective was perhaps somewhat different but also reality-based. (See Chapter 5.) In the process and through friends in Washington, we met with the staff at Columbia and with Dr. Barry Gurland. I was happy to discover that there were other people in New York who were as concerned as I was about what was not going on in this field, in this state and the reasons why.

In the intervening years, and it is three years now since that began, I have visited a great many organizations throughout the country. I have been pleased with most, have read much of the existing literature (which does not take long) in this field and come to the conclusion that what we needed to do was to accomplish it ourselves. As a result, we are breaking ground in Dutchess County for a life-care type of community in New York. I stress that most strenuously because we have tried with the help of some of the conference participants, particularly Aaron Rose of Laventhol and Horwath and others to wend our way between the rules, regulations and pitfalls that we anticipated in New York State. It certainly has been a frustrating procedure. But I realize that we are not alone. There are somewhere in the state, in one form or another, people who have done the same. Some have been grandfathered because their communities have existed in some form for many years. Others have very quietly done what they had to do and hidden their talents under a bushel in the hope that they would escape all the laws of New York.

Despite the myths about relocation, over two-thirds of the retired civil service workers in the state elect to remain living in New York State and do not flee to Florida. The state with an aging population now finds it advisable to provide tax forgiveness for those retired over the age of 60-1/2 in order to encourage them to remain in the state. In view of the fact that nursing home beds are virtually frozen, or might as well be, the state is developing rules and regulations to encourage home health care and home nursing care. However we still do not have a clear path to providing for many people the kind of living and the kind of care that they are seeking.

To explore the possibilities of change and to determine where change was advisable, we decided to hold a conference inviting people with considerable experience in the area of continuing care retirement communities. The chapters that follow cover the areas which were subjects of the conference though not necessarily presented in the order in which they appear in this volume.

ORGANIZATION OF THIS VOLUME

With the exception of Chapter 2, this volume is composed of papers presented at the conference as well as of condensed reports on the conference workshops which dealt with the legal, social, financial and policy issues related to the conference theme. Included also is a portion of an Executive Summary which was produced by Dr. Paul Wagner and the NPO/Task Force Inc. staff for distribution to state officials, legislators, conference participants and other interested persons.

Part I contains a socio-historical overview of the concept of continuing care as well as a nation-wide survey of existing financial and legal regulations of the industry.

Part II discusses the legal, financial and ethical implications of continuing care communities.

Part III moves from the general to the specific case study of a continuing care retirement village in Pennsylvania.

Part IV contains 3 papers by New York State officials commenting on the historical background of current State policies and speculating about the future establishment of continuing care retirement communities in New York State.

Part V includes condensed workshop reports dealing with existing conditions and barriers in New York State and proposing solutions and recommendations for future action.

Part VI reproduces the narrative portion of the Executive Summary of the conference concluding with an Epilogue.

PART I:
CONTINUING CARE
RETIREMENT COMMUNITIES:
AN OVERVIEW

Introduction to Part I

This section contains two papers that deal with the concept and definition of continuing care communities. In *Chapter 1*, Laurence Lane introduces the concepts of compact and contract in the original social context of a community that assumes the responsibility of caring for and sharing with its members. He then relates how changing circumstances forced the informal compact of early continuing care communities to evolve into a more formal contract that covered all aspects of rights and responsibilities between consumers and providers. Although the *paper of Chapter 2* was not presented at the conference, we asked the publisher's permission to reprint it for inclusion in this volume. Sarah Williams, editor of the Alpha Centerpiece, offers a clear definition of Life Care. Her report also covers the issues of financial risks and the need for regulation which are being discussed in the following chapters of this volume.

1

Chapter 1

Continuing Care—Consumer Choice: From Compact to Contracts

Laurence F. Lane

This chapter addresses the developing service approaches to the elderly in the context of the "new paternalism versus laissez-faire capitalism."[1] Historically, the communal approach to sharing and caring constituted an informal compact among members of a community. Changes, often external to service delivery, forced the formalization of care agreements. Such formal protection to the consumer have altered the nature of service delivery and changed the attitudes of providers.

First, the evolution of formal service agreements will be traced and then their substance will be described. It is possible that the formalization of agreements between the providers and consumers has undermined the potential communal position of continuing care retirement communities. This issue merits attention inasmuch as a contract significantly affects the relationship between residents residing in such a community and the sponsoring provider entity.

The concept of community is deeply rooted in the 19th Century.[2] Beginning with Hegel and spanning most of the great macrotheorists of the 19th century the writings of that period were a response to the "problems of order created at the beginning of the nineteenth century by the collapse of the old regime under the blows of industrialism and revolutionary democracy."[3]

The nature of the community was carefully scrutinized in a search for stability. Most writers of the 19th century developed typologies with which to classify communities and some contrasted stable, homogeneous communities of previous historical periods with the

Laurence F. Lane is Director for Non-Proprietary and Special Programs, American Health Care Association, Washington, D.C.

3

volatile, heterogeneous communities in which they lived and/or contrasted the urban environment with rural lifestyles. The contrast which Tonnies drew between the "Gemeinschaft" and "Gesellschaft" type of relationships[4] is not dissimilar from the distinction between the community-based service provider mechanism represented by the ideal continuing care community and the contrasting public contract for shelter and services from nursing homes developed as an offshoot of federal domestic policies since the 1930s.

It is relevant to point out that the community initiatives of the Progressive Era, which are at the root of the nonprofit delivery system of services to older persons, were developed in quest to reclaim the traditional values of the Gemeinschaft-type of environment. They were in direct contrast to the public almshouse approach of the late 19th century and they have survived the Gesellschaft-type policies of the 20th century to this day. Their survival has been sustained primarily because of the emotional and financial support of communities which sponsor such institutions.[5] It can be argued that the formalization of the contractual agreement utilized by continuing care communities alters the "shared risk" to which the general community of residents have agreed and thereby weakens the chances of continued survival by voluntary homes.

Two distinct theories of alienation emerged from the 19th century writings which are the basis of modern day sociology and psychology. One viewed the root of alienation as being conditioned by society and the other saw it as a problem of the individual.[6] Both theories provide valuable insights into understanding why religious and fraternal communities took initiatives to establish institutions to serve "their own members" and why individuals sought to pursue such voluntary attachments with specific communities.

In any discussion of an appropriate role for government in policing the behaviors of providers of continuing care, we must be explicit as to our values with respect to community. The legacy of old age homes is one of providing a Gemeinschaft-like environment for residents in a world which has come to accept Gesellschaft-like requirements because they reflect a norm.

Stripped of all its financing and service delivery characteristics, the continuing care agreement constitutes a shared promise. Individuals make a promise to share their wealth with others and providers make a promise to provide necessary services. Trust becomes the primary bond which holds the agreement together. Under conditions of certainty, the ability of both parties to fulfill the agreement is greatly assured. Under conditions of uncertainty, keeping the promise becomes much more difficult.

A number of changes have increased the probability of uncertainty in care delivery. Such changes as those itemized below have eroded the idea of a compact between provider and resident and established the course toward a formalized contractual relationship. The following list is far from exhaustive.

Economic uncertainties—depressions, recessions, inflation and other business cycle changes have greatly complicated the ability of the provider to calculate the cost of services. It is sometimes hard to remember that before the Great Depression that began in 1929 the Eagles and other non-profit fraternal organizations had turned homes for the aging into a mature industry. The depression undermined the abilities of families to provide supplements for care and services and also changes in the Old Age Assistance portions of the original Social Security Act provided a disincentive to placement.[7]

Changing demographics—declining mortality rates have greatly complicated the certainty of providing care and services: the young old may not need it; the old old may need more than a community can provide.

Service approach changes—the past fifty years have witnessed tremendous changes in types of services provided. The homes for the aged of fifty years ago were primarily social care facilities providing shelter, congregate dining and protective oversight. It has been only during the past three or four decades that such facilities "medicalized" their service delivery.

Changing expectations—not only has the service approach changed, the public perception of what a facility-based program for the elderly should provide has greatly changed. There are public expectations for staffing levels, types of amenities, recreational opportunities and service delivery. Each increment of service adds to the costs. Each cost adds to the problem of pricing for future services.

Changing public requirements—not only have the expectations of the consuming public changed, so have the rules imposed by public agencies. As I have written in other articles, among the most significant factors in the long term care delivery system have been the physical plant safety requirements and especially the fire safety codes imposed by government action.[8] Other changes, including changes in the minimum wage requirements and standards for licensure have added to the costs of providing future services.

Changing technology—while long term care facilities have not been affected to the same extent as hospitals, technology has affected costs. The report of the Committee on the Future of the American Association of Homes for the Aging released last year suggests that changing technology may have a tremendous impact on the pricing of long term care services, especially where there is a commitment of current dollars for future services to be provided in the coming years.[9]

Changing business approaches—providing for long term service needs has generated a long term care industry in the marketplace. Managing and owning have become the norm for the industry rather than sponsoring and serving. The business of long term care has become very formal; the portion which provides continuing care has followed suit. The informal sense of sponsoring support for a community has been replaced by explicit statements of liability.

The typology of living arrangements developed by Joyce Parr for the Foundation for Aging Research[10] identifies the various changes made by facilities to accommodate these external influences. The Foundation for Aging Research study documents a number of different directions taken by providers to respond to these changes. The development of a full-service retirement community is only one of a range of options pursued by providers. (There may be some advantages to relaxing the rigid definition of continuing care retirement communities employed in the Wharton School study[11] to permit consideration of other service approaches which are financed through a continuing care payment.)

As noted above, the formalization of the obligation between the continuing care provider and the consumer has taken many forms. The spectrum runs from cryptic admissions agreements to nearly unreadable legal contracts. There are no standardized contract forms used in the profession. Moreover, it is more the norm than the exception for a provider to have several different contracts to offer prospective residents. While examples of a compact arrangement can still be found, most homes now have established a written agreement which can be construed as a contract. The actual impetus for a formal contract has been in response to state regulations, i.e., state licensure requirements, taxation revenue rulings and spend-down provisions for the Medicaid program.

Howard Winklevoss has described the financing of a continuing care retirement community in Chapter 3. One of Winklevoss' key observations is that a home confronts a ''gross liability which is divided into group liability and individual liability.''[12] A contract is a form of dividing this liability. The following are general areas of formal agreement which have been observed in continuing care retirement communities contracts:

Defining services, coverages and accommodations—Hackler has written, "the kinds of services and medical care that are to be provided under life care contracts need not be the problems that they now are. A properly drawn contract can set out what is to be provided by the home and what is expected from the residents."[13] One of the primary admonitions in the *Guidebook for Consumers: Continuing Care Homes* (Published by the American Association of Homes for the Aging) is that "the contract you sign should describe the type of shelter and services covered under the payment schedule listed in the contract."[14] Ann Trueblood Raper in her analysis of data for the AAHA Continuing Care Retirement Community Survey has provided a useful summary of the services found in the over 200 communities responding to the survey.[15] Harvey Pies has identified the following six areas as the most important coverage areas: "(i) hospitalization, (ii) transfer to nursing home facility, (iii) physician services, (iv) registered nurse services, (v) exclusions and areas of non-coverage, and (vi) apartment features."[16] One point needs to be emphasized in discussing services, coverages and accommodations: there has been a proliferation of approaches; thus the prospective resident should shop around to see which of the various packages meets his needs.

Defining fees—"Before signing a contract for continuing care," the AAHA Consumer Guidebook exclaims, "you should clearly understand the home's charges and the methods by which you will be expected to pay for the shelter and services you receive."[17] The data analysis developed for the University of Pennsylvania study indicates a range of entrance fees from $1,000 to $187,000 with an average fee of $35,000. The same data indicates a monthly fee of between $300 to $1,000. An article written by David Cohen advocates greater scrutiny of financial management of homes citing, "the unique financial dynamics of a continuing care community" as "particularly vulnerable to quite innocent miscalculations."[19] In his checklist to providers for life care contracts (Figure 1) Hackler includes the following provisions: "(i) state fees to be charged, both endowment fees and monthly fees, and (ii) provide for increase in monthly fees."[20] In spite of such advice, the Winklevoss Study indicates that 27% of the communities still have a limit on monthly fee increases.[21]

Admissions—The data analysis from the University of Pennsylvania Study conducted by Winklevoss and associates indicates that most communities have a requirement that individuals must be over a specified age before entering the facility. Nearly two-thirds of the communities also require minimal levels of assets and require a minimum level of monthly income. More than half of the communities studied mandate medical insurance in addition to Medicare. Six out of ten communities are certified for Medicare and fifty percent use Medicaid.[22]

Termination—The AAHA guide notes "it is important that you know in advance under what circumstances the home can discharge residents or transfer residents to other accommodations."[23] The data from the University of Pennsylvania study indicates that over

Figure 1

CHECK LIST—LIFE CARE CONTRACTS

This is a checklist for life care contracts. It is not intended to be an all encompassing guide to life care contracts, however, it will highlight the problem areas outlined above and give you an indication of the quality of your present contract.

1. State services and facilities to be provided.
2. State Medical, Nursing Home, or Hospital Care provided.
3. State Fees to be charged—both Endowment Fees and Monthly Fees.
4. Provide for increase in Monthly Fees.
5. Require that rules and regulations be followed subject to change.
6. That representations in Application by resident are true.
7. Reserve corporation's right to determine admissions and dismissals.
8. Reserve right to change accommodations for residents.
9. Resident shall provide his own clothing or other items.
10. No responsibility for loss of property.
11. Corporation should have right to enter resident apartment.
12. Provide for disposition of property or removal on demise of resident.
13. Provide for resident's inability to handle personal affairs.

Figure 1 continued

14. Reimbursement of corporation by injury or damage by negligence by resident.
15. Lien for Medical Care in event of negligence of Third Party.
16. Rights of parties upon termination of Agreement.
17. Prohibit Assignment of contract rights to third person.
18. Disclaimer—only the written contract is binding.
19. Waiver of one breach not a waiver of any other breach of contract.
20. Right of Management to operate the home reserved to corporation.
21. Residents agree to apply for government funds.
22. Financial ability—no resident discharged by reason of inability to pay is discretionary with Board and provided no transfer of assets by resident.
23. Loss of tax exemption clause.
24. Laws of the state where home situated to control contract provisions.
25. Right of Resident is not proprietary interest in properties or assets of corporation.

Hackler, Eugene, "Legal and Practical Aspects of Life Care Contracts," Hackler, Londerholm, Speer, Vader and Austin, 201 N. Cherry Street, Olathe, Kansas. (unprinted and undated manuscript)

two-thirds of the homes have stipulations which permit contract termination.[24]

Transfer—Another area of importance is the grounds under which an individual can be transferred from his apartment to another accommodation. Many facilities have a clause in their general rules and regulations which empowers the management to impose case management. About half of the homes have a specific contract provision which mandates that an individual who requires transfer give up his apartment if he cannot return to it within a certain period of time, generally somewhere between thirty and ninety days.[25]

Refunds and probationary period—One of the areas of greatest change has been with respect to refund policies. When the AAHA Consumer Guide was written seven years ago, a small percentage of communities permitted a probationary entry and refund. Now, about half permit a probationary entry and most provide for some refund policy under specified conditions. The liberalization of refunds has given rise to the refundable life fee approach which has been experimented with in some areas and with the notion of a pre-paid capitation approach to services with a declining balance. Potential residents should carefully review the options which are available. Often, there is a need to weigh the initial pricing of services, with coverages and refunds.

Property rights—Recent years have seen an evolution of the approaches taken by providers with respect to granting property rights to residents. The argument advanced in the *Onderdonk* case in New Jersey is characteristic of the traditional view, "what is abundantly clear from the very beginning of continuing care contracts as they have evolved over 200 years is that residents in continuing care homes are *not* tenants."[26] The court upheld the argument denying plaintiffs relief under the state's Anti-Reprisal Act. However, some continuing care programs have been initiated which utilize a "condominium and/or cooperative" approach which separate the service components from the living arrangement. These creative initiatives often concede specified property rights in return for permissive rules to apply case management assistance to residents, i.e., the right to transfer and/or expell an individual. Prospective residents of a full-service community should be conscious of the opportunities to retain specified property rights.

Rights of collective representation—Considerable attention has been given in recent years to the value of resident councils and other means of resident participation in the governance of the community. A contract should be scrutinized to ensure that the rights for collective representation are not abridged.

Contractual rights are probably only as useful as their enforcement; thus, there has been an increased emphasis on the policing of provider behavior. While David Cohen touches on several aspects of the enforcement process in chapter 4 and mentions others in his earlier paper,[27] there is merit in restating briefly his views. Four, generally complementary, approaches have been tried:

State statutes—Nearly a dozen states have enacted specific continuing care statutes. While the form of the statutes vary, most provide for state certification of the continuing care provider; full disclosure to the resident by requiring approval of promotional materials, contracts, and financial conditions; financial requirements for putting entrance fees into escrow during construction, the mandating of specified audit and lien requirements; and establishing a procedure for addressing conflicts.[28] One of the intriguing results of state requirements for continuing care has been the establishment of a "franchising" right which works to the advantage of current providers and adds legitimacy to the care approach. New York must decide whether the fledgling "underground" continuing care industry which is circumventing the existing state rules merits attention.

Provider self-policing—The exchange of information stimulated by the University of Pennsylvania study has been facilitated by a desire on the part of many providers to "police" the practices of the industry. Certainly, during my years of working with the American Association of Homes for the Aging it was clear that every effort was being made by the provider community to be responsive to changing public expectations of performance. One group in the Delaware Valley has been very successful in utilizing an accreditation approach. Unfortunately, as we have learned from recent legislative debates on the survey and certification rules suggesting changes in the Federal regulations to permit "deemed status" review by the Joint Commission on the Accreditation of Hospitals, public opinion toward long term care facilities is negative towards the idea of self-policing.

Resident self-governance—Considerable attention has been given to expanding the role of the residents in governing CCRC's. David Cohen seems to be a strong proponent of such reforms as a means of ensuring provider responsiveness. While not questioning the merits of such participation, there are a number of practical questions which arise in balancing power-sharing with current residents vis-à-vis the abilities of an organization to serve future residents. There are taxation complications if the facility takes on the appearance of cooperative.

Informed consumers—In testimony before the Senate Special Committee on Aging, Commissioner Patricia Bailey of the Federal Trade Commission commenting on the FTC's investigation of a life care organization remarked, "The Commission is hopeful that the affirmative disclosures required by the order will provide beneficial and important information for prospective residents of all life care homes."[29] Affirmative disclosure requirements are the central component of many state statutes on life care. Information published by interest groups serving life care providers and by providers themselves have emphasized the need for careful consumer review of all aspects of the care program before commitment. Perhaps the most significant change of the past century with respect to this care approach has been that the compact based on trust has sometimes been unfulfilled. Disclosure of practices and state action to police misinformation have strengthened the ability of consumers to shop around for the best programs for their needs.

At the beginning of this chapter, there was a question as to whether the change from a compact to a contract has benefitted the consumer. Amitai Etzioni in the *Active Society* makes a powerful case for developing authentic institutions. "Authenticity exists," he points out, "where responsiveness exists and is experienced as such . . . authenticity requires not only that the actor be conscious, committed and hold a share of the societal power, but also that the three components of the active orientation be balanced and connected."[30] Perhaps the real strength of the continuing care community approach is its potential to sustain an authentic response to the needs of a portion of our aging population. Contracts have become the instrument for ensuring a balance. They have also become an instrument for informing the public of the abilities of a provider to meet their needs. Thus, it is critical for the consumer to carefully compare the offerings of several communities before making a choice. And it is critical for the consumer to play an active role in the community of his choice.

REFERENCE NOTES

1. American Society of Law and Medicine, "Legal and Ethical Aspects of Health Care for the Elderly," a workshop conducted in Washington, D.C., June 2-4, 1983.

2. Lane, Laurence F. "Healthy Remnants of an Earlier Era: Continuing Care, A Differing Policy Perspective," American Association of Homes for the Aging, January, 1979.

3. Nisbet, Robert A. *The Sociological Tradition* (New York, Basic Books) 1966, p. 21.

4. Tonnies, Ferdinand. "Gemeinschaft and Gesellschaft," as cited in Warren, Roland, *New Perspectives on the American Community* (Chicago, Rand McNally, 3rd Ed.) 1977, p. 11.

5. Lane, *op. cit.*

6. Isreal, Joachim, *Alienation from Marx to Modern Sociology, a Macrosociological Analysis,* (Boston; Allyn & Bacon) 1971, p. 139.

7. For a good discussion of the impact of the New Deal see: Thomas, William, *Nursing Homes and Public Policy,* (Ithaca, NY; Cornell University Press) 1969.

8. Lane, Laurence F. "The Nursing Home: Weighing the Investment Decisions," *Hospital Financial Management,* May, 1981.

9. American Association of Homes for the Aging, *The Report of the Committee on the Future: A Working Draft,* Washington, D.C., October, 1981.

10. Parr, J. and Green, S. *Housing Environments of Elderly Persons: Typology and Discriminant Analysis,* (Clearwater, FL; Foundation for Aging Research), 1981.

11. Continuing Care Retirement Community Study, The Wharton School of the University of Pennsylvania, 1981-1983.

12. Winklevoss, H.E. and Powell, A., "Retirement Communities: Assessing the Liability of Alternative Health Guarantees," *Journal of Long Term Care Administration,* 1981.

13. Hackler, Eugene, "Legal and Practical Aspects of Life Care Contracts," unpublished, Hackler, Londerholm, Speer, Vader & Austin, Olathe, Kansas, c. 1980.

14. American Association of Homes for the Aging, *Continuing Care: A Guidebook for Consumers,* Washington, D.C., 1976.

15. Raper, Ann Trueblood, "Continuing Care Retirement Communities Data Analysis Report," American Association of Homes for the Aging, Washington, D.C., March 1982 (performed as part of the Continuing Care Retirement Community Study, The Wharton School of the University of Pennsylvania, 1981-1983.)

16. Pies, Harvey, "Life Care Communities and Residence Care Agreements," presentation to the conference on Legal and Ethical Aspects of Health Care for the Elderly, American Society of Law and Medicine, June 4, 1983.

17. AAHA, *Continuing Care: A Guidebook for Consumers, op cit.*

18. Raper, *op. cit.*

19. Cohen, David, "Continuing Care Communities for the Elderly: Potential Pitfalls and Proposed Legislation, *University of Pennsylvania Law Review,* 1980.

20. Hackler, *op. cit.*

21. Raper, *op. cit.*

22. *Ibid.*

23. AAHA, *Continuing Care: A Guidebook for Consumers, op. cit.*

24. Raper, *op. cit.*

25. *Ibid.*

26. *Paul T. Onderdonk, et al., vs. The Presbyterian Homes of New Jersey, Inc, et al.,* Supreme Court of New Jersey, C-461 September Term 1979, Docket No. 16, 788.

27. Cohen, *op. cit.*

28. "State Legislation Regulating Continuing Care Homes," *Continuing Care: Issues for Nonprofit Providers,* American Association of Homes for the Aging, Washington, D.C., 1980.

29. Senate Special Committee on Aging, "Testimony of Commissioner Patricia P. Bailey concerning Life Care Homes," May 25, 1983.

30. Etzioni, Amitai, *The Active Society* (New York; Free Press) 1968, Chapter 21, p. 621.

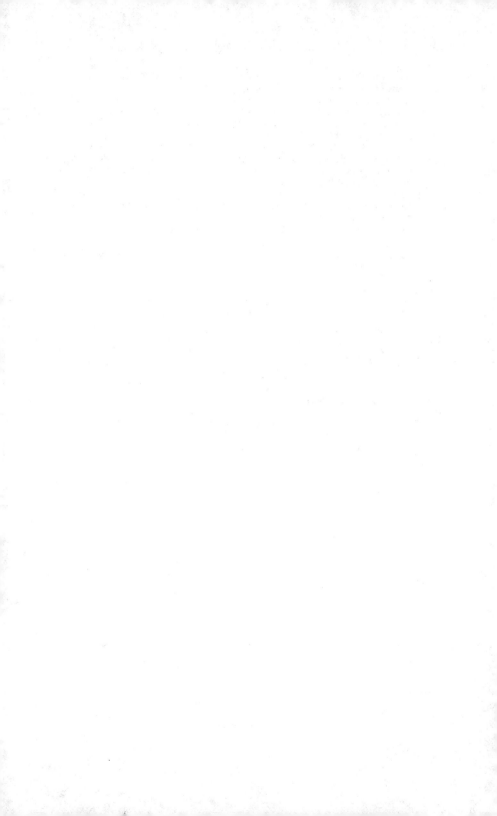

Chapter 2

Long-Term Care Alternatives: Continuing Care Retirement Communities

Sarah Williams

ABSTRACT. Definition of Life Care Community. A continuing care requirement community (CCRC), or life care community, is a long-term care alternative providing a package of services, including housing, health care and social services, to the elderly. More specifically, a CCRC: (1) provides independent living units, either apartments, rooms or cottages; (2) guarantees a range of health care and social services, which may include intermediate or skilled nursing care, usually available on the premises; (3) requires some type of prepayment, generally an entrance fee and/or monthly fees; and (4) offers a contract that lasts for more than one year or for life and that describes the service obligations of the community and the financial obligations of the resident.

One of the most critical problems facing states today is the escalating cost of long-term care for their elderly citizens. In 1982 state and local governments paid $7.1 billion in total nursing home expenditures. With the aging population growing at a rate three times faster than that of the general population, the cost of caring for the elderly will continue to rise rapidly in the years ahead. In an effort to slow this steady increase in costs, many states are looking at new ways to finance long-term care for the elderly.

But cost is not the only concern. State policymakers are now rec-

Sarah Williams is Editor of the Alpha Centerpiece, Alpha Center, Bethesda, Maryland.
The Alpha Center is partially supported by the Health Resources and Services Administration under contract HRSA 232-79-0035. Statements made in this publication do not necessarily represent the policies or viewpoints of the United States Government.
15

ognizing that adequate long-term care means more than nursing home care; it involves a coordinated system of health care, social services and housing. To meet this need, a number of states are also considering innovative models for long-term care that provide a total package of services to the elderly.

One approach gaining in popularity is the continuing care retirement community (CCRC), sometimes referred to as the life care community. This alternative to the nursing home and other forms of long-term care is increasingly attractive to many elderly because it guarantees them lifetime care, as well as housing and other services. Proponents of the concept also envision life care as affordable for a large proportion of the aging population despite the widespread view that it is a viable option only for the well-to-do. A new comprehensive study of CCRCs, prepared for the Wharton School of the University of Pennsylvania,* concludes that the majority of elderly citizens have the financial means to pay for life care.

The very nature of the life care arrangement, however, brings with it serious financial risk, not only for the community and its developers, but especially for the residents. For this reason the Wharton School study calls for state regulation of the industry to ensure careful financial planning of CCRCs and to protect the financial security of their elderly residents.

The focus of this issue of *Alpha Centerpiece* is the role of the states in the development of life care communities. A number of states have already adopted programs to regulate the life care industry; others are still studying CCRCs to determine whether they should encourage or discourage their development. To assist states in this review, we examine here the advantages CCRCs offer and their potential for mismanagement and fraud that can result in financial disaster. We also describe some of the steps states can take to protect the residents of CCRCs. Finally, we look at existing regulatory programs in general and in selected states.

Future issues of *Centerpiece* will discuss other delivery and financing alternatives for long-term care, including capitation financing

---

Continuing Care Retirement Communities: An Empirical, Financial, and Legal Analysis, by Howard E. Winklevoss and Alwyn Powell, published for the Pension Research Council, Wharton School, University of Pennsylvania. The study was funded jointly by the Commonwealth Fund and the Robert Wood Johnson Foundation. Copies are available from the publisher, Richard D. Irwin, Inc., 1818 Ridge Rd., Homewood, Illinois 60430, (312) 798-6000.

models (social/health maintenance organizations) and hospital-based programs.

LIFE CARE DEFINED

The concept of life care was developed to meet the elderly's need for an independent way of life, and to give them the security of guaranteed, affordable health care and other services. Life care is generally regarded as a kind of social and health insurance plan for the aging.

Life care facilities or continuing care retirement communities vary widely in their financing arrangements, in the type of housing available and in the range of services provided. Consequently, a variety of definitions exists. Similar to other kinds of nursing homes and congregate housing for the elderly, they provide independent living units, such as apartments or cottages, and they offer various social, recreational, maintenance, and health care services, usually on the premises. In exchange for these services, residents pay a substantial fee.

But the distinguishing feature of the CCRC, as defined here (see box on page 2), is the continuing care or life care *contract*. Under terms of the contract, which lasts for more than one year or for life, the community promises to provide housing, health care and various services, and the resident agrees to pay, in advance, certain fees to help cover the cost of these services. Although the fees cover the cost of housing, these payments do not give the resident any owner-ship rights.

The earlier life care communities required residents to turn over all of their assets in return for lifetime shelter and services. Today most communities require payment of an entrance fee and a monthly service charge. According to the Wharton School study, the average entrance fee in 1981 was $35,000, with 80 percent in the range of $13,000 and $65,000; the monthly fee averaged $550, with most communities charging between $300 and $900. CCRCs usually vary their monthly fees on the basis of the type of housing selected and the number of occupants in each unit.

As with any type of insurance plan, the advanced funding for future services provides the financial foundation of CCRCs. The community pools the revenues it collects from residents, including entrance fees, monthly fees and Medicare, Medicaid and private insurance payments. Although residents selecting similar units will pay similar fees, the cost of providing services to them will vary since some will live longer than others and some will require more nursing care. In principle, the excess costs incurred by these residents will be covered by the reserved pool of funds received from others who need fewer services.

Life care communities are generally selective in admitting elderly individuals. Residents usually have to be a certain minimum age, have a minimum level of assets, have no pre-existing serious health problems, and be covered by Medicare and private insurance plans. The result of this selective admissions policy is that CCRC residents tend to be healthier and wealthier than the elderly in the general population.

Although a number of communities were established before the 1960s, most of them have been constructed in the last 20 years. Today there are about 300 CCRCs in the United States, according to the definition used by the Wharton School. The American Association of Homes for the Aging (AAHA) also lists about 300 in its directory of life care communities to be published in January, but other groups, using less rigid definitions, have estimated as many as 600. Estimates of the number of persons housed in CCRCs range from 55,000 to 100,000.

Life care communities are found throughout the United States, but are most concentrated in states with large elderly populations: California, Florida, Pennsylvania, Ohio and Illinois. An exception is New York, which despite its large number of aging citizens, prohibits the development of life care facilities.

The first communities were organized and sponsored by religious and charitable organizations. Today the majority are owned by nonprofit corporations, still mostly church-related groups. Only about 5 to 10 percent of CCRCs are owned by for-profit institutions. But as many as a third of the communities sponsored by not-for-profit groups are being managed by outside proprietary companies, the Federal Trade Commission reports.

PROSPECTS FOR GROWTH

In recent years high interest rates have slowed the development of CCRCs. Not only has it been difficult for developers to raise the necessary capital for construction, but potential occupants have had trouble selling their houses to obtain money for the entrance fees. But with declining interest rates and increased real estate sales, the number of new communities is expected to grow rapidly in the decade ahead. The Philadelphia accounting firm, Laventhol & Horwath, predicts that an additional 1,000 to 1,500 communities will be in operation by 1990.

ADVANTAGES TO ELDERLY

Even with the predicted growth of the life care industry, only about 2 percent of the elderly are expected to reside in CCRCs by 1990. But proponents of life care see the communities as an attractive option for an even larger share of the growing elderly population. They offer certain advantages that other long-term care arrangements cannot provide. Life care represents an alternative to institutionalization for older people who can no longer maintain their own homes for both health and financial reasons, but who do not want or need the extensive care provided in a nursing home. Unlike nursing homes and other retirement communities, CCRCs give their aging residents the assurance they can live independently as long as possible and they can receive nursing care and support services as long as needed.

Another benefit of CCRCs is that the quality of care may be better than in other types of long-term care facilities. Studies have shown that the residents of life care communities live 20 percent longer than the elderly population at large. They also tend to use health care resources less than the residents of comparable facilities. These favorable health status factors may be attributed to the availability of prepaid health care and other community services; they may also be influenced by the self-selection process, which reflects the better health and higher income of those choosing CCRCs.

The major advantage of life care, however, is that it is affordable to most elderly Americans, contrary to the widespread notion that only the wealthy can afford the fees. The range of fees charged by CCRCs is "within the financial grasp of the majority of individuals over age 70," the authors of the Wharton School study concluded. This may be especially true for the older communities, which have paid off most of their debts and can therefore charge lower fees.

Since most elderly own their own homes, they can usually raise enough cash from selling their houses to pay the entrance fees.

Social security and private pension benefits are generally sufficient to cover the moderate and relatively fixed monthly service charges. In approximately 54% of the communities the monthly payment remains the same when the resident is transferred to the nursing facility. The monthly rate at a comparable nursing home outside the community could be considerably higher.

ADVANTAGES TO FOR-PROFIT COMPANIES

Another reason for the expected increase in the number of CCRCs is that the expanding elderly population, with its financial assets, offers new business opportunities for the proprietary institutions. Although most CCRCs are owned and operated by non-profit groups, an increasing number are under the management of for-profit corporations. In addition, more and more proprietary firms are becoming interested in developing life care communities because of the opportunities for profits and income tax savings.

As pointed out by Laventhol & Horwath in its 1982 report on the life care industry, land sales, developers' charges, construction contracts, marketing fees and management contracts can all produce profits, and depreciation of real estate investments can result in tax benefits. Among those for-profit concerns looking into the opportunities to be found in the life care business are architects, construction firms and real estate developers, as well as proprietary nursing homes and hospitals, the accounting firm said.

FINANCIAL RISKS

While the concept of life care promises financial and social security for many elderly Americans, it also poses significant financial risks. Some experts estimate that at least 10 to 20 percent of existing CCRCs have experienced financial difficulty or are in danger of developing serious fiscal problems in the future.

The danger lies in the considerable potential for mismanagement and fraud inherent in the unique contractual relationship between the life care community and its residents. If a community runs into financial difficulty, because of poor financial planning or fraud, it may not be able to fulfill its commitment to the residents. The residents, having already fulfilled their part of the bargain by committing much, if not all, of their assets to the community, may be left with nothing: no shelter, no health care and no money.

Potential for Mismanagement

The potential for financial management problems exists because of the complicated financing required to develop, construct and operate a life care community. Without careful planning and application of sound actuarial principles, a community may be doomed to failure.

Crucial to a CCRC's financial solvency is its ability to calculate accurately the residents' fees, which are used to cover current and future capital and operating costs. CCRC managers must project the costs of future health care services for the residents and then establish a pricing policy to fund that obligation, Howard Winklevoss, principal author of the Wharton School study, pointed out. They must also anticipate the costs of renovating and replacing the physical plant. Possibilities for making innocent errors during the price-setting process abound.

Mistakes are often made in projecting the resident population in the years ahead, estimating the number of deaths and the number of transfers to the nursing facility. When a resident moves to the nursing facility, the vacated apartment becomes available to a new resident, who will pay a new entrance fee. When a resident dies, the community now has unlimited access to any remaining entrance fee. This reliance on turnover is a concern to some critics of the life care concept, who see it as a disincentive to care for residents. But turnover of residents is essential to financial success and is the basis of establishing fees. Failure to use morbidity and mortality tables that adjust for the healthier CCRC population can result in an overestimation of the turnover rate and the setting of lower fees and consequently, lower revenues than expected.

Another problem is failure to maintain adequate reserves. Reserve funds are needed to protect against lower turnover in the beginning and unpredictably low turnover rates in the future, as well as unforeseen capital and operating costs, high inflation rates, and the inability of residents to meet payments. Some communities may be tempted to overspend in the early years when their operating costs are low and their revenues high from the accumulation of entrance fees, attorney David Cohen, a collaborating author on the Wharton School study, pointed out. Later, when the health of the residents declines, costs will increase as additional nursing care is required. The community then may not have sufficient funds in store to cover these subsequent costs because of excessive spending earlier.

A third common error is a reluctance to raise the monthly fees to make up for earlier miscalculations in the rate structure, Cohen wrote in a 1980 *University of Pennsylvania Law Review* article. Sometimes a community that initially charged high entry and low monthly fees may find it necessary to raise the monthly charge in order to increase revenues. Residents on fixed incomes, however, may not be able to afford the higher fees. In the past some CCRCs have prohibited or limited increases in a resident's monthly payments. But if a financially distressed community "either cannot or will not raise its monthly fees quickly enough to make ends meet, the result is financial disaster," Cohen concluded.

Potential for Fraud

The potential for fraud in the life care industry exists merely because of the community's receipt of large entrance fee payments—perhaps totalling millions of dollars—in the early years of operation, before expenses mount up. During this period, a fraudulent operator could divert this money to its own use rather than setting it aside to pay for the future costs of caring for the community's residents. When the time comes to provide skilled nursing care to the residents, there may not be enough money to pay for it. Some observers believe that the likelihood of fraud has increased with the growing involvement of for-profit institutions in the operation of life care communities.

The best known example of fraud is the case of Pacific Homes, a chain of life care facilities sponsored by the Methodist Church. In 1977, Pacific Homes declared bankruptcy after incurring a deficit of $27 million. This financial dilemma was the result of the diversion of substantial cash prepayments from community residents for "expansion, speculative investments and payment of current operating losses," said the report of the bankruptcy trustees. In order to pay for the care of the residents whose funds had already been spent, the corporation had to sell more life care contracts. "The scheme continued so long as enough new people could be induced to enter into the contracts," the report concluded. Nearly 2,000 elderly people were affected by the bankruptcy.

Inadequate Disclosure

In addition to the financial risks inherent in a life care contract, residents may be at risk because of a community's failure to provide full disclosure of its financial status. In some cases the information given to a prospective resident may not be adequate for a reasonable judgment about whether to enter into a contract. In other cases, including examples uncovered during federal investigations, the information about the community's financial condition may be intentionally misleading. One common deception found was false representation about religious affiliation, leading potential residents to believe wrongly that some church entity would bail out the community in the event of financial difficulty.

NEED FOR REGULATION

Because of this potential for mismanagement and fraud, most observers believe that some form of regulation is needed to ensure the financial viability of life care communities and to protect the welfare of the residents. The question is whether such regulation is the responsibility of the federal government or of the states.

Limited Federal Role

So far the federal government's involvement in life care has been limited mainly to Medicare and Medicaid certification requirements for CCRC nursing facilities. Federal legislation regulating certain aspects of the life care industry has been proposed in the last few years, but no action has been taken.

Last May, the Senate Special Committee on Aging held a hearing on life care communities, with one panel of witnesses describing the advantages CCRCs offer to the elderly and another panel discussing some of the problems. The committee has not yet developed a legislative position, but it is concerned with the inadequacy of some state regulations to protect the residents in case of financial failure, said David Holton, the committee's chief investigator. One legislative approach being considered, he said, is to establish certain federal criteria for life care communities; CCRCs in states with regulations satisfying the criteria would be exempt from federal requirements.

The Federal Trade Commission began investigating the marketing and managing practices of the life care industry in 1978 in response to complaints from residents of several communities. As a result of that investigation, the FTC took action last summer against Christian Services, Inc. (CSI), a proprietary corporation involved in the management of more than 50 life care facilities in 17 states. The major thrust of the FTC's order was to require adequate disclosure to prospective residents of the financial risks involved in contracting for life care. Other provisions prohibited misrepresentations, such as false or misleading statements about the role of the mortgage lender, service fee increases, or religious affiliation. CSI was also required to issue statements disclosing the nature of any reserve funding, the intended use of prepaid entrance fees, and the disposition of any reserves for projects unrelated to the community. Many of the provisions in the order were drawn from the disclosure requirements in existing state laws and a model bill developed by AAHA.

The FTC's order applies only to CSI, but the commission regards it as "a statement of expectations" for all life care communities, even for nonprofit facilities beyond FTC's jurisdiction, said Henry Whitlock, staff attorney in charge of the investigation. Any community not in compliance with the order's provisions could be subject to action by the FTC, he warned, and other enforcement agencies could take action against any nonprofit facility.

State Regulation Favored

Rather than a federal law for life care communities, state legislation is generally regarded as the most appropriate way to regulate the industry. The Wharton School study concluded that it would be better to encourage a variety of state legislative programs than to enact a broad federal statute since CCRCs are still relatively new and differ widely from region to region. So far 10 states have adopted comprehensive legislation and about six have programs aimed at only one specific aspect of the industry. In a few other states, legislation is under consideration.

After discussing in detail the provisions contained in existing state statutes, the Wharton School study described the elements that should be included in any state regulatory program. The first requirement is for a definition that would bring all types of life care communities within the scope of the law. The definition should include communities charging an entrance fee and/or monthly fees, and should cover contracts lasting for more than a year, or for life, as well as mutually terminable agreements. Second, the study recommended that states adopting continuing care legislation require certification of all communities before they can open for business. But approved private self-accreditation programs could perform the certification functions for the state, the authors added.

To protect the residents' investment, the study called for two types of entrance fee escrows, one for existing and operating communities and another for new communities, with provisions specifying how and when the funds would be released to the operators. Any state legislation should mandate the maintenance of actuarially sound reserve funds, but the study did not recommend a specific level.

Other recommendations related to the residents' relationships with the community. First, states regulating CCRCs should require communities to file annually a complete financial disclosure form with the administering agency and to give prospective and current residents a simplified disclosure form, with a clear narrative description of the community's financial condition. States should also require submission of all advertising and promotional materials for approval by the agency. In addition, the study recommended a provision guaranteeing the residents' rights of self-organization.

Finally, every statute should contain detailed investigative and enforcement authority provisions, the study said, but should not mandate rehabilitation of financially-distressed communities by outside parties.

Self-Accreditation

For some, self-accreditation is seen as a way to ensure quality in the life care industry without the expense and burden of regulation. The Continuing Care Accreditation Association, headquartered in Pennsylvania, has reviewed and accredited 12 facilities in the Delaware Valley, according to Lloyd Lewis, chairman of the association's board. Lewis is also executive director of the Quaker-affiliated Kendal Crosslands, which operates two communities in the Philadelphia area. The current focus of the accreditating group's review, said Lewis, is on the financial solvency of a community and the adequacy of its disclosure policy. In the future, the group hopes to expand its review program to include New England and other regions.

Lewis believes such a peer review program is more effective than a law; it can also save money in administration if accredited facilities are exempt from certification requirements, as is proposed in the Pennsylvania legislation (see below). The Wharton School study also recommended that CCRCs receiving accreditation from an approved program should be exempt from certain statutory certification requirements. This approach is similar to Medicare's reliance on the Joint Commission on the Accreditation of Hospitals' (JCAH) standards.

Others, however, are more skeptical of the ability of self-policing programs to protect residents of life care communities. For example, during recent legislative debates on the JCAH review process, several groups representing the aging strongly opposed any self-accreditation in the long-term care industry.

CURRENT STATE APPROACHES TO REGULATION

So far 10 states have adopted comprehensive legislation regulating the life care industry: Arizona, California, Colorado, Florida, Illinois, Indiana, Maryland, Michigan, Minnesota and Missouri. Although specific provisions vary from state to state, all the laws include a definition of the entity to be regulated and requirements covering certification, financial status, relationships between residents and communities, and state administration.

Definition

The definitions of CCRCs in the state laws are so diverse that some communities regulated in one state would not be regulated in another. Generally the definition describes the regulated community by the terms and duration of the contract, the types of services provided and the financing arrangements. Some states, such as California, Florida and Illinois, include communities charging an entrance fee or monthly fees, or both. But the definition in Arizona, for instance, covers only communities with an entrance fee, leading some CCRCs to change their policies and require only large periodic payments in order to escape regulation.

Certification

All states require some type of a preliminary registration and certification by a state agency before a community can sell a contract and begin operation. Only Florida requires provisional certification prior to full certification. Procedures for certification generally spell out the kind of financial information to be submitted to the agency so it can assess the financial stability and integrity of a prospective operator. Provisions on renewal and revocation of certification are also included.

Regulation of Financial Status

All laws include various provisions designed to ensure the financial solvency of CCRCs and protect the residents if financial problems do develop. One such provision is a requirement that a resident's entrance fee and deposit be placed in escrow until he moves into the unit, with varying formulas for release of the escrow funds. In addition to this entrance fee escrow, most states require CCRCs to maintain reserves to protect against potentially difficult financial periods in the future. The composition and minimum levels of the funds differ widely as do restrictions on investment of the reserves. A few states also authorize the administering agency to require a surety bond to protect residents.

Regulation of Resident-Community Relationships

Public disclosure of financial information is required by all the states, although the type of information to be disclosed is not always the same. Some states permit the general public and prospective and current residents to inspect the financial statements and annual reports submitted to the administering agency. Most require communities to furnish prospective residents with copies of specific materials to enable them to evaluate the community's financial condition before signing a contract. The majority of state laws also include some form of advertising regulation.

To further protect prospective residents, most states regulate to some degree the form and content of the life care contract. California, Colorado and Florida require approval of the contract by the agency. These states, as well as Illinois and Maryland, have detailed contract requirements, covering such provisions as the community's rates and the type, cost and duration of the services to be provided. Some laws also require the contract to state the health and financial status residents must maintain to stay in the community. Most statutes have refund provisions, with some requiring a full refund of prepayments if a resident dies before occupancy. Many refund provisions allow prospective residents to cancel their contract during a certain "cooling off" period, and a few provide for dismissal of a resident by the community under certain conditions.

Only three states, Florida, Michigan and Missouri, give residents the right to self-organization so that they can have a voice in the management of the community and can be kept informed on community affairs. Finally, six states require CCRCs to give their residents a lien or preferred claim to protect them from total financial loss in case of insolvency.

State Administration

The agency responsible for administering the program varies among the states. Four states have designated the insurance department as the administering agency; the social services, securities and public health departments and the aging office have been selected in other states. Minnesota has no administering agency because its law is self-executing. A number of states also have advisory councils to help the agency in implementing the program.

Most states grant their agencies some level of authority to investigate and inspect CCRCs. In terms of enforcement authority, some laws authorize injunctive relief against violations of the law, some grant a cease and desist power, and all provide civil and/or criminal penalties for violations by individuals. Finally, if a community gets into serious financial difficulty, the agencies of six states are authorized to take over the community's management under certain conditions in order to rehabilitate it.

SELECTIVE STATE REGULATION

A few states have decided to regulate only specific aspects of the continuing care industry rather than to enact detailed, extensive legislation. For example, Connecticut has a law limiting the eligibility of life care residents to receive Medicaid benefits. Similar restrictions had been adopted in Illinois before it passed its comprehensive life care act in 1982. Legislation enacted in Oregon in 1977 requires a life care community to refund any entrance fees or down payments to a resident who withdraws from the facility during the first six months of occupancy.

In an effort to encourage the development of CCRCs, other

states, including New Jersey, have adopted regulations that exempt community nursing home beds from certain certificate of need (CON) requirements (see below). Florida has a similar CON policy for CCRC long-term care beds, although it also has a comprehensive law regulating the life care industry, unlike New Jersey.

LEGISLATION UNDER CONSIDERATION

In addition to these states with legislation on the books, several more are considering proposals to regulate the industry. One of these is Pennsylvania, where a bill passed the Senate and awaits action by the House early in 1984 (see below). A number of other states have established task forces to review legislative options and recommend regulatory approaches.

Those seeking long-term care alternatives in New York are also interested in legislation on life care communities, which are currently prohibited in the state. Under regulations adopted in 1969, no nursing home operator can enter into a "life care" contract or accept prepayment for "basic services" for more than three months. Concerned that many elderly retirees are moving to other states that offer life care, the Columbia University Center for Geriatrics and Gerontology held a conference last June to study whether CCRCs should be encouraged in New York. The consensus of that conference was that the state should open the door for the development of CCRCs. Specific recommendations included changing the rules to permit life care arrangements and developing legislation to guard against financial failure of communities. As a result of the conference, the New York Association of Homes for the Aging is working with the legislature, state officials and other groups to explore legislative and regulatory options for the life care industry.

The following examples show how three different states—Florida, New Jersey and Pennsylvania—are dealing with the life care industry.

FLORIDA

Florida has a special need for long-term care alternatives because of the state's Medicaid policy, according to Karen Torgesen of the Florida Association of Homes for the Aging (FAHA). Many elderly people cannot afford the average monthly charge of $1,500 for nursing home care yet their income is too high to qualify them for Medicaid. For them, life care communities represent an affordable option, particularly one of the many older, nonprofit facilities with entrance fees in the range of $8,000 to $15,000.

Because of its large population of elderly, the largest in the country, Florida is a prime market for the development of CCRCs. There are about 60 communities now, with applications pending for 20 more, Torgesen said. But many of these proposed projects will never get off the ground because they will not meet the requirements of the state law, she said.

The first law, passed in 1954, covered only facilities that charged initial prepayments and no monthly maintenance fees. Close to 95 percent of the communities developed during this period required only a monthly payment so they escaped regulation, Torgesen explained. Then in 1977, after a decade of financial troubles and bankruptcies in the industry, the state passed a new statute with strict reserve provisions and complicated administrative procedures. The definition included both communities charging entrance fees and those charging monthly fees. Amendments adopted in 1979 and 1981 further expanded the definition to include facilities providing personal care services rather than nursing care. These revisions added even more stringent reserve requirements.

In response to continued financial difficulties, the legislature made additional changes in 1983, based on the recommendations of an advisory panel composed of representatives of the legislature, the Department of Insurance, the long-term care industry and consumer groups. The amendments were designed mainly to improve financial planning by requiring proof of a proposed project's financial feasibility before construction or operation can begin, and to protect against future fiscal problems by increasing the level of reserve funds.

Unlike other states, Florida requires provisional certification of prospective CCRC operators by the Department of Insurance, the administering agency. The application must include organizational and construction data, financial information, advertising samples, a copy of the contract, disclosure of conflicts of interest, and a preliminary feasibility study. Receipt of a provisional certificate entitles a provider to collect entrance fees and/or deposits, which must be placed in escrow until the department authorizes release.

Once an operator has a provisional certificate, it can apply for a certificate of authority, which is required for operating or constructing a facility or issuing continuing care agreements. The application must include additional financial information and a final feasibility study. Under a unique provision in the 1983 amendments, the applicant must also show that the project has at least 50 percent of the units reserved, with the provider having collected a minimum of 10 percent of the entrance fees charged for each unit. Two percent of the entrance fee is not refundable except upon the death or serious illness of a prospective resident or for other reasons beyond the control of the operator. This provision is designed to prevent prospective residents from paying the minimum deposit during the project's planning state, and then later demanding their money back, leaving the facility with insufficient funds to finish the project.

In addition to the entrance fee escrow provision, the Florida law requires a reserve fund escrow to protect communities during difficult economic periods. The new amendments raise the required reserve level to equal the total amount of all principal and interest payments due during the fiscal year on any mortgage loan or other long-term financing, including taxes and insurance. Half that amount was required before. Existing facilities are given 20 years to comply.

The Florida statute mandates full financial disclosure to current and prospective residents, including information on all ownership interests and lease agreements. It requires departmental approval of the contract and specifies its form and content, including the terms and conditions under which an agreement can be canceled and the entrance fee refunded. Florida goes further than other states in recognizing residents' rights to self-organization, allowing them to choose their own representative and to engage in concerted activities, and requiring quarterly meetings between residents and management to discuss the facility's financial status and proposed changes in policies and services.

In terms of administration, the Florida legislation allows the department to inspect a facility's records at any time but requires examination every three years. It also provides for injunctive relief for violations and civil or criminal penalties for violations by individuals. Finally, the statute authorizes the department to take over the management of a facility in serious financial difficulty under certain conditions.

NEW JERSEY

Although New Jersey has considered legislation regulating the life care industry, it has not yet adopted a comprehensive regulatory program. But last May the New Jersey Department of Health did adopt an amendment to its CON regulations designed to encourage the development of CCRCs as an alternative to nursing homes. The revision, which became effective June 6, 1983, exempts CCRC on-site nursing facilities from certain CON review criteria, if the following conditions are met:

— the community has a minimum of 200 residential units;
— the ratio of residential units to long-term care beds is not less than 3.3 to 1; this ratio is in line with the 60 bed unit size already required for nursing homes;
— within five years of occupancy of the first apartment, at least 70 percent of the nursing facility's occupants will be drawn exclusively from the life care community; and
— long-term care patients who are from the general population are allowed to stay as long as they need to, "regardless of the number of residents who are waiting for long-term care services."

If a CCRC meets all of these criteria, its proposed long-term care beds will not be counted in the bed need for the health planning area. Further, the community nursing facility may be exempt from utilization criteria and batching cycle requirements. Instead of the long, involved CON review process required for other types of nursing facilities, the CCRC's application may be subject to an expedited administrative review under which the HSA staff can make a recommendation directly to the Department of Health, bypassing two additional levels of review.

While the state has an overall excess of nursing homes beds, a shortage exists in some areas, where the elderly complain of long waiting lists to get into nursing facilities. The exemption from the area bed need count was established because a CCRC's long-term care beds are used primarily for its residents, and do not compete directly with free-standing nursing home beds, explained John Sunkiskis in the state CON program office. In the early years of operation when residents are generally healthy, a community must usually let outsiders use its nursing facility in order to generate revenues.

But later, when the health of the residents deteriorates, most of the nursing bed occupants will come from the CCRC.

So far the department has approved the nursing facility proposals of four communities, with a few more meeting the criteria, Sunkiskis said, Because of the growing interest in life care as a long-term care alternative, he expects to see many more in the future.

In addition to the new CON policy, other actions in the state point to a favorable environment for CCRC development, according to Laurence Lane, a policy consultant on services for the elderly. One is a recent change in regulations on industrial revenue bonds, making it easier for homes for the aging to get tax-exempt financing. The publication this fall of the Wharton School study, funded in part by the Princeton-based Robert Wood Johnson Foundation, is also expected to give a boost to life care communities, he said. Finally, New Jersey's potential market for CCRCs may be enhanced by the current restrictive policy in neighboring New York.

PENNSYLVANIA

The life care industry flourishes in Pennsylvania despite a 1975 nursing home regulation prohibiting residents from turning over all of their assets in return for life care. According to the Pennsylvania Association for Nonprofit Homes for the Aging (PANPHA), there are about 30 communities in the state, most of which are in the Philadelphia area. The majority of these CCRCs, as in other states, require an entrance fee and monthly payments. Although there have been cases of financial difficulty and fraud in Pennsylvania, at present the communities are not regulated.

But a comprehensive bill patterned after the AAHA model statute and drafted chiefly by the state association, is close to enactment. The proposal passed the Senate last July and is now awaiting final action in the House early in 1984. Life care legislation had been considered in 1982 following Senate investigative hearings on the CCRC industry and a report by a Senate-convened task force of health care and legal consultants.

According to its definition of continuing care, the bill now before the state legislature would cover only communities requiring payment of an entrance fee, with or without a monthly charge; communities charging high monthly fees and no entrance fees would be exempt from regulation. Mutually terminable contracts are specifically included. Like all other states, the bill would require a facility to be certified before it may operate. But unlike other legislation, certification requirements would be waived if a facility is accredited under a private program approved by the Department of Insurance, the administering agency.

Before a prospective resident signs a contract, a facility would have to provide a disclosure statement, including information on the corporate structure, ownership interests and any outside management arrangements; a description of the services to be provided and the fees required; and detailed financial information.

The bill also contains provisions aimed at protecting a community's financial standing. It would require each provider to maintain reserves in an amount at least equal to the total of all principal and interest payments due during the next year, or 10 percent of the projected annual operating expenses, whichever is greater. As further protection in certain cases, the department could require a provider to have a reserve fund escrow. In addition, the bill would mandate an entrance fee escrow, with separate formulas for release of the funds, depending on whether the residential unit is new or old. The proposal would also provide liens if deemed necessary by the department.

Other provisions in the bill specify the content of the contract, such as descriptions of the services and the terms governing refunds, in clear, understandable language. Like the Florida law, the bill would also recognize the right to self-organization and would require quarterly meetings between residents and the management.

Finally, the proposed legislation would grant the department rehabilitative authority, and investigative, audit and subpoena powers. It would also provide for injunctive relief and criminal and civil penalties for violations of the law.

PART II: LEGAL, FINANCIAL AND ETHICAL ISSUES

Introduction to Part II

The three papers in this section deal with the legal, fiscal and ethical implications that are inherent in the establishment of continuing care retirement communities in this country in general as well as in the state of New York in particular. In *Chapter 3*, David Cohen discusses the currently existing approaches to legal regulation of CCRCs as they exist in the United States, i.e., comprehensive statutory legislation, non regulation and limited regulation (which is the case in New York). He points out that in his opinion regulation is necessary to assure the quality of CCRCs. *Chapter 4* deals with the financial issues that must be considered in relation to existing and future continuing care communities. Howard Winklevoss who, with his associates at the Wharton School of the University of Pennsylvania did a survey of 270 CCRCs, touches briefly on the important issues of actuarial reserve, income accounting principles and professional fiscal management needed for CCRCs. He also stresses the need for the development of an industry-wide data base and future research in the areas of morbidity, mortality and health services utilization within those communities. Monsignor Charles Fahey, in his address reproduced in *Chapter 5*, is concerned about the ethical aspects of policies which would support the establishment of CCRCs in New York State. He wants to make sure that there are enough safeguards in place to protect consumers and providers alike from potential failures and hardships.

35

Chapter 3

Legal Regulations
of the Continuing Care Retirement
Community Industry as a Whole

David L. Cohen

This chapter describes in relatively general terms some of the more technical aspects of legal regulation of the life care or continuing care industry.

Three different areas are covered. First, there is a description about what exists around the country in terms of regulation of the continuing care industry. Second, some apprehensions are reported about the state of the law in New York, New Jersey, and Connecticut. Finally, there is a general discussion about why regulation is important and why it appears to be something with which we either fortunately or unfortunately have to be concerned.

There are three approaches to regulation of the continuing care industry around the country.

The first approach concerns a brief description (though the list of references contains a number of works giving greater details) of the extensive regulation of continuing care communities. A set of regulations called ''Life Care Community Regulation'' (not Medicaid regulation) to which life care communities might have to comply, is certainly detailed and extensive. In this category fall ten states: Arizona, California, Colorado, Florida, Illinois, Indiana, Maryland, Michigan, Minnesota and Missouri. For some reason, the alphabet stops just before New York. (See charts at the end of this chapter, summarizing the Status of Current Legislation.*)

David L. Cohen is Associate in the Philadelphia Law Firm of Ballard, Spahr, Andrews & Ingersoll.

*These charts were prepared in connection with the Continuing Care Retirement Community Study, Wharton School of the University of Pennsylvania, 1982.

37

These states have relatively comprehensive statutes that contain a number of specific types of regulatory provisions. Some are listed below in order to illustrate what is meant by extensive regulation. A typical comprehensive statute might provide some or all of the following kinds of regulatory controls: certification of provider, escrow requirements, reserve requirements, financial disclosure, lien and preferred claim provisions, provisions requiring surety bonds to be posted for the security of the community, detailed regulation of the form and content of the continuing care agreement itself, advertising regulation directed specifically at the continuing care industry, a detailed investigative, enforcement, and rehabilitative mechanisms for communities. In one way or another this might move outside the statutory scheme.

The second approach is nonregulation. A response which has been adopted by thirty-six states, the District of Columbia, and the federal government. This statement should be qualified because it really is not fair to call it nonregulation. Much activity is going on even in states that do not regulate continuing care communities.

Parenthetically it should be added there are many states that should not even be thinking about regulating continuing care communities. Roughly thirty states out of the fifty have three or fewer continuing care communities presently operating. It seems clear that if, for example, the state of Nevada does not have any life care communities, it should not spend a lot of time worrying about passing a comprehensive statute regulating what is a nonexistent industry. So the statement: "there are thirty-six states, the District of Columbia and the federal government that are doing nothing" is not meant to be critical. There are three states that have many life care communities. Even though they are not presently regulating the industry, they are considering doing so. The three states that fit into this category are: New Jersey, Ohio, and Pennsylvania. By 1984, it will be probable that Pennsylvania also will have a comprehensive statute regulating life care communities.*

New Jersey's efforts are also worth viewing because it is a direct neighbor of New York. In 1981, then Assemblyman Snedeker introduced a comprehensive statute regulating the continuing care industry. Apparently, nothing happened. Because Assemblyman Snedeker is no longer in the legislature, nothing is going on in New Jersey at this time.

---

*In fact, Pennsylvania has recently adopted a comprehensive statute regulating the continuing care industry. (Editor's note.)

In addition, the federal government's role in regulation should be mentioned. At present, it has an inactive role. A number of people who have contributed to this volume or who participated in the conference on which it was based, were involved in the first congressional hearing in May 1983 on the life care industry in Washington. Probably no legislation will come out of that hearing. The hearing appeared to have been an overview and investigatory hearing of what is going on. However, it appears that some attention is being paid in Washington and life care communities are not a case of abject neglect.

The final category of the present regulatory environment may be labeled as limited regulation. Two forms of limited regulation should be mentioned before getting to the case of New York. First, there is the regulation that exists in the State of Oregon, which regulates the refund mechanism of life care communities.

A digression is necessary in order to describe the Oregon statute because it is unclear where it came from. Right in the middle of a nice, beautiful book of statutes there is one paragraph that says: if a resident of a life care community dies within six months of moving into a life care community, he/she gets back his/her full entrance fee. It was difficult to understand why that paragraph was inserted. Last year, at a meeting in Atlanta, when this was pointed out, somebody from Oregon explained that the speaker of the Oregon state house had a favorite junior high school teacher who was living in a life care community and died within six months of moving in. Her heirs were very upset that they did not get any of her money and came running to him. He said, "Oh, that's awful!" and introduced the legislation.

There is a lesson to be learned from this episode. That is, the legislation probably causes no harm because it is not clear how many life care communities there are in Oregon but it is a bizarre statute and it or something like it might turn up elsewhere.

The second form of limited regulation is present in Illinois and Connecticut. The easiest way to summarize that is by a statutory codification of what you will read in Part II concerning the New York State regulatory provision of Medicaid eligibility for life care residents. The Connecticut statute was struck down by a three-judge federal court and the United States Supreme Court as being violative of the supremacy clause of the Constitution on the grounds that it is unconstitutional for a state to *presume* the availability of assets of the community to a resident. Now this is not to say that the Connecticut law is not on the books, but there is a United States Supreme Court decision which says that statute cannot be enforced. It is not clear whether Connecticut is enforcing the statute or not. Nor is it clear whether on the basis of that authority, the Illinois Department of Public Welfare stopped enforcing the Illinois statute, although the Illinois statute itself is also still on the books.

This leads to New York's response to life care which is really the second part of this chapter. Chapters 8, 9 and 10 explain what the New York regulations say and theorize about how this came to be. Some of the arguments bear repeating and they will be discussed here in a slightly different way. The N.Y. State regulations prohibit any residential health care facility operator from accepting pre-payments for basic services for more than three months or from entering into any life care contract. That seems to mean three different things: first, the most likely explanation is that New York has intended to and has in fact prohibited life care, continuing care, and anything that looks like life care or continuing care, with an entrance fee up front and a monthly payment.

That is not to say you cannot have anything someone might call life care in New York. For example, there can be grandfathering provisions. Another example is something that the firm with which I am associated has become very involved with in Florida, not New York, and that is, a splitting of the residential and health aspects of the life care community. No prepayment, just monthly pay as you go in the residential part, monthly pay as you go in the medical part and all you have in common is ownership and a common campus. You still have the sense of community but you do not have the insurance aspect of community care.

It should be added that there is an incidental benefit to this type of structure from the development perspective. When you structure your community in this way, you have made yourself partially eligible for FHA insurance. If you are eligible for FHA insurance and you go the tax exempt bond route, you get a better rating on your tax exempt bonds.

Now, the second way you could look at the N.Y. State regulation is to say that it does not mean what it says. However, an alternative interpretation should be considered. This interpretation is as follows: what New York was really trying to do was prohibit life care, that is, what we would call life care. By life care, we do not mean a contract for an entrance fee and a monthly fee that stays the same. By life care, we mean Pacific Homes style life care. That is what was around when New York enacted its regulation. The Pacific

Homes style of life care represented the following three patterns: (1) a resident turns over all his money and the community takes care of him for the rest of his life (it is understandable why New York might not want to let anyone get away with that); (2) a resident has a little money and it is not fair to take all of his money; thus the resident is asked to turn over X dollars and in exchange the community will take care of him for the rest of his life and will charge a monthly fee. This position also raises problems; (3) a resident turns over X dollars and pays X amount per month which will never change. The monthly fee will never be raised. In exchange the community will take care of him for the rest of his life.

The three patterns listed above are pure forms of life care, and it appears that the New York regulations clearly were intended to preclude any operator from offering a life care contract. Contrast that with continuing care, if you will, as we know it today. Continuing care in most states is where there is an entrance fee that might change over time for different residents coming into the community, where the entrance fee through accounting mechanisms might be able to be allocated exclusively to capital expenditures as opposed to basic services, and where there is a monthly fee that adjusts over time for inflation which is paying for basic services. Thus, the monthly fee becomes a payment for basic services for which there is no prepayment.

In concluding it is necessary to say that there is some support for that type of interpretation of N.Y. State's regulations. The Pennsylvania nursing home regulations provide support for that type of interpretation. Pennsylvania has the third largest number of continuing care retirement communities in the country. It has thirty-one of them. And on the books in Pennsylvania, right now, in black and white is a regulation that says that no residential health care facility operator shall offer a contract for life care. It is not known whether anyone ever went in and argued with the Pennsylvania Department of Health about what its regulation meant. However it is clear that a regulation worded almost precisely the same way as New York's has absolutely no effect in deterring the development of an industry barred in New York, just 120 miles to the south of New York. So, there is some support for the second interpretation of N.Y. State's regulations. However, this should not be misconstrued to mean that it might be advisable for anyone to run out and build a continuing care community without doing a lot more work on the subject.

Regulation is important and the way a state's regulation looks will affect very substantially the quality of the industry that develops in that state. This is asserted for the following reasons: (1) if you have good regulations you can increase certainty in this industry. For example, if you have regulation, and by regulation is meant statutory regulation, it says in black and white you can have a contract that does not have a refundable entrance fee. As long as you disclose that it is not a refundable entrance fee, you will not have a lot of lawsuits claiming it is unlawful to have nonrefundable entrance fees. Lawsuits are very expensive. Thus it is necessary to increase certainty in that area; (2) another reason for regulation is to increase the certainty that a community will survive. One of the things discussed throughout the process of writing up the Wharton School study, and Howard Winklevoss deals with this in the following chapter is the reserves issue. If you have adequate reserves, you do not have to worry about a community going under. And if you do not have to worry about a community going under, that solves just about all the problems everyone is concerned about.

Now, one of the things we played around with is the notion of an actuarially sound reserve. And, although the study did not come straight out and recommend this, a number of people who worked on it individually believed that ten years from now that is where we should be. That is, a statute is not going to say that you have to have a reserve of X dollars or of sufficient dollars to cover X obligations, but rather that you have to have a reserve which some kind of an outside expert—an actuarial consultant, an accountant, an underwriter—says is adequate.

The days are over when one was able to say regulation is not needed and communities can do just fine on their own. There are not too many states with large numbers of communities which are going to permit that mind to govern anymore. And, if that view no longer obtains, then one has to think about what belongs in legislation or regulation and what does not belong. Those judgements will certainly affect the quality of the industry. Who are you going to have in the industry? Is it going to be small church-related providers or is it going to be the multi-state nursing home chain?

Regulation and the shape of regulation is really a crucial issue for consideration in the years to come. The bottom line seems to be that this industry belongs. The safest thing to do is to make the decision that it is a good idea to protect consumers—and it might be added to protect operators from themselves as well—and say "yes we should do that." But the best way to do that is to get rid of a regulation which purports to prohibit continuing care and make it clear that it is not the industry which is prohibited but unwise practices. Thus the industry needs to be regulated in order to make it safe.

CHARTS SUMMARIZING THE STATUS OF CURRENT LEGISLATION*

TABLE 1

DEFINITIONS

Arizona	California	Colorado
Contract to provide for a person for life or for a term in excess of one year medical services and board and lodging conditional on payment of an entrance fee in addition to or in lieu of periodic payments.	Contract to provide for a person for life or for a term in excess of one year medical service and board and lodging conditional on payment of an entrance fee in addition to or in lieu of periodic charges including continuing care agreements.	Care provided under a contract for life of an aged person including health care and board and lodging.

Florida	Indiana	Maryland
Furnishing of nursing care, shelter, and food upon payment of an entrance fee. Continuing care shall include only life care, care for life, or care for a period of one year or more.	Contract to provide for a person for life or for a term in excess of one month medical services and board and lodging conditional on payment of an entrance fee in addition to or in lieu of periodic payments.	Furnishing for money care or shelter to an individual over age 60 under a contract with (1) required 12 or more months of care to another to be paid in advance; (2) provide for care for more than one year; or (3) provide for life care.

Michigan	Minnesota	Missouri
Three part definition covering only life care and care for more than one year. Labels the former "life interest" and the latter" long term lease."	Furnishing to an individual of board and lodging together with medical services pursuant to a written agreement effective for the life of the individual or for a period in excess of one year.	Furnishing shelter, food, and nursing care to an individual for life or for a term of years. Care for a term of years defined to include care in excess of one year and an agreement for continuing care for an indefinite term.

AAHA		
Agreement for the payment of an entrance fee and/or periodic charges in exhange for living accommodations, medical care, and related services which is effective for the life of the individual or for a period in excess of one year.		

*These charts were prepared in connection with the Continuing Care Retirement Community Study, Wharton School of the University of Pennsylvania, 1982.

TABLE 2

CERTIFICATION

PROVISIONAL CERTIFICATION

Arizona	California	Colorado
None.	None.	None.

Florida	Indiana	Maryland
Required application with attachments. Then can collect entrance fees and enter into feasibility study.	None.	None.

Michigan	Minnesota	Missouri
None.	None.	None.

AAHA

None.

CERTIFICATION

Arizona	California	Colorado
Can't sell contract without certification.	Can't sell contract without certification.	Can't sell contract without certification.

Florida	Indiana	Maryland
Required for operation.	Can't sell contract without certification.	Can't sell contract without certification.

Michigan	Minnesota	Missouri
Can't sell contract without certification.	Can't sell contract without filing (self-executing statute).	Can't sell contract without certification.

AAHA

Can't sell contract without certification.

TABLE 3

FINANCIAL INFORMATION REQUIRED

Arizona	California	Colorado
Balance sheets, income statements, and projected income statements.	Past 3 years balance sheets and income statements plus 5 year projections.	Certified financial statements and projected income statements for at least a five-year period.

Florida	Indiana	Maryland
Use of proceeds statements plus balance sheet and income statement. Also, computation of debt service requirement and information on plant equipment and property.	Financial statement of the provider prepared in accordance with generally accepted accounting principles.	Certified statement of applicant's financial condition.

Michigan	Minnesota	Missouri
Balance sheet, use of proceeds statement, and feasibility study.	Balance sheet and income statements. Projected income statement for next year.	Comprehensive financial statements with specifics varying depending on whether the CCRC is new or old. Also statement of reserve and escrow provisions.

AAHA

Certified financial statements and income statements. Projected income statements for next year.

TABLE 4

RENEWALS, REVOCATIONS, ETC.

Arizona	California	Colorado
Annual filings, but certification valid unit revocation.	Annual filings, but certification valid until revocation. Independent revocation procedure.	Annual renewal procedure. Independent revocation procedure.

Florida	Indiana	Maryland
Annual renewal procedure. Independent revocation procedure.	Annual filings, but certification valid until revocation. Independent revocation procedure.	Annual renewal procedure. Independent revocation procedure.

Michigan	Minnesota	Missouri
Annual renewal procedure. Independent revocation procedure.	Annual filings, but certification valid until revocation. Independent revocation procedure.	Annual renewal procedure. Independent revocation procedure.

AAHA

Annual filings, but certification is valid until revocation. Independent revocation procedure.

TABLE 5

ESCROW PROVISIONS

Arizona

Entrance fee escrow until occupancy for new units. Complicated formula for release of funds. Also requires a reserve fund escrow equal to aggregate principal and interest payments due on first mortgage over next 12 months.

California

Entrance fee escrow until oocupancy for new units. Simple formula for release of funds. Also requires a reserve fund escrow equal to aggregate interest, principal, and lease payments due over next 12 months, if accommodation fee exceeds 100 times the monthly fee.

Colorado

Entrance fee escrow until occupancy for new units. Complicated formula for release of funds. Also requires a reserve fund escrow equal to 65% of all large sum initial payments. This reserve is to be amortized over the first five years of residence, but at no time is the reserve to fall below 35% of the original requirement.

Florida

Entrance fee escrow required until certification and obtaining of long term financing. Also requires a reserve fund escrow equal to aggregate of one-half the principal interest and lease payment due over the next fiscal year.

Indiana

Entrance fee escrow until occupancy for new units. Complicated forula for release of funds.

Maryland

Entrance fee escrow required until certification.

Michigan

Entrance fee escrow until occupancy for new units. Special provision authorizing state to require an escrow of a reasonable amount when financial conditions become precarious.

Minnesota

Entrance fee escrow until occupancy for new units. Complicated formula for release of funds. Also requires a reserve fund escrow equal to aggregate of principal and interest payments on first mortgage due over next 12 months.

Missouri

Entrance fee escrow until occupancy of new units. Complicated formula for release of funds. Also requires a reserve fund escrow equal to 50% of any entrance fee paid by the first occupant of the unit. This reserve is to be amortized and "earned" at the rate of one percent each month. But the reserve never can fall below 150% of the annual long term debt principal and interest payments of the provider.

AAHA

Authorized the department to require an entrance fee escrow until occupancy. Complicated formula for release of funds.

TABLE 6

SIZE

Arizona

Total of interest and principal payments due over the following year on account of any first mortgage or other long term financing of the facility.

California

Total of interest, principal, and rental payments due during the next year (same as Arizona plus rental payments). Also a requirement that reserve be sufficient to cover the obligations assumed under continuing care agreements, as calculated through the use of state approved mortality tables.

Colorado

65% of the amount of any advance payment made by all residents. Straight line amortization over a 5 year period. At no time can reserve fall below thirty percent of the original requirement.

Florida

Amount equal to one-half the aggregate amount of all principal and interest payments due during the fiscal year on any mortgage or other long term financing on the facility, including taxes and insurance and leasehold payment.

Indiana

None. Has a Retirement Home Guarantee Fund instead.

Maryland

None.

Michigan

None.

AAHA

None.

Minnesota

Amount equal to the total of all principal and interest payments due during the next 12 months on account of any first mortgage or on account of any other long term financing of the facility.

Missouri

Requires a reserve fund escrow equal to 50% of any entrance fee paid by the first occupant of the unit. This reserve is to be amortized and "earned" at the rate of 1% each month. But the reserve never can fall below 150% of the annual long term debt principal and interest payments of the provider. Plus each CCRC must establish a reserve equal to at least five percent of the facility's total balance of contractually obligated move-out refunds at the close of each fiscal year.

TABLE 6, continued

INVESTMENT LIMITATIONS

Arizona

Must be placed in "escrow," but the principal of escrow account may be "invested," apparently without limitation with the earnings and up to 1/6 the principal payable to the provider. Principal released to the provider must be repaid within 2 years.

California

The former reserve requirement must be placed in escrow, but the funds can be invested with the same limitations as apply to the second type of reserve. These limitations allow investments in bank deposits, first mortgages, approved bonds and stocks, real estate, furniture and equipment of the community. 25% must be in cash and listed bonds and stocks. If the community has at least half its contracts on a monthly basis, only 5% need be in these liquid investments.

Colorado

Reserves must be held in bank accounts, first mortgages, real estate, or furniture of the community. At least 10% must be in bank accounts and listed bonds or stocks.

Florida

Subject to general investment limitations imposed on insurance companies with provision for emergency release of funds to the provider.

Indiana

None. Has a Retirement Home Guarantee Fund instead.

Maryland

None.

Michigan

None.

Minnesota

Must be placed in "escrow," but the principal of the escrow may be "invested," apparently without limitation with the income and 1/12 of the principal payable to the provider.

Missouri

Must be placed in "escrow" but can be held in federal government or other marketable securities, deposits, or accounts insured by the federal government.

AAHA

None.

TABLE 7

BONDING REQUIREMENTS

Arizona	California	Colorado
None.	Agency may require a bond in any reasonable amount when necessary to protect the residents. Fidelity bond also required.	None.

Florida	Indiana	Maryland
None.	A community may replace entrance fee escrow requirement with a letter of credit	None.

Michigan	Minnesota	Missouri
Agency may require a bond in any reasonable amount when necessary to protect the residents.	None.	None.

AAHA

A community may replace entrance fee escrow requirement with a surety bond.

TABLE 8

FINANCIAL DISCLOSURE TO RESIDENTS

Arizona

Furnish copy of latest
annual report to pro-
spective residents
before signing of
contract.

California

Furnish financial state-
ments to prospective
residents before signing
of contract.

Colorado

Furnish copy of latest
annual report to pro-
spective residents
before signing of
contract.

Florida

Allows public inspec-
tion of reports filed
with the state. Must
post a summary of latest
examination report and
latest annual report in
facility. Disclosure of
same to prospective
residents.

Indiana

Allows public inspection of
reports filed with the state.
Furnish copy of latest
annual report to prospective
residents before signing of
contract.

Maryland

Allows public inspection
of filings.

Michigan

Allows public inspection
of filings.

Minnesota

Detailed financial dis-
closure to prospective
residents before signing
of contract.

Missouri

Furnish copy of latest
annual report to pro-
spective residents
before signing of
contract. Annual dis-
closure.

AAHA

Detailed financial dis-
closure to prospective
residents before signing of
contract. Annual disclosure.

TABLE 9

CONTRACT REGULATION

SUBMISSION TO STATE

Arizona	California	Colorado
No.	Submit and approve.	Submit and approve.
Florida	Indiana	Maryland
Submit and approve.	Submit only.	Submit only.
Michigan	Minnesota	Missouri
No.	Submit only.	Submit only.

AAHA

No.

DETAILED REQUIREMENTS

Arizona	California	Colorado
No.	Yes.	Yes.
Florida	Indiana	Maryland
Yes.	No.	Yes.
Michigan	Minnesota	Missouri
No.	No.	No.

AAHA

No.

TABLE 9 continued

REFUNDS

Arizona	California	Colorado
Not addressed.	Must have refund of admission fee less reasonable expenses within 10 days of cancellation. Does not deal with contingency of death.	Must have refund of difference between amount paid in and the amount used for care of the resident. Special provision for tax-exempt CCRCs.
Florida	**Indiana**	**Maryland**
Full refund if resident dies before occupancy. All refund provisions must be stated in contract. Must be within 120 days and on a pro-rata basis. Contingency of death must be addressed.	Not addressed.	Full refund if resident dies before occupation. All refund provisions must be stated in contract. Contingency of death must be addressed.
Michigan	**Minnesota**	**Missouri**
Full refund if resident dies before occupation.	Full refund if resident dies before occupation.	Not addressed.

AAHA

Not addressed.

TABLE 10

RIGHTS OF SELF-ORGANIZATION

Arizona	California	Colorado
None.	Regulation grant right to form a residents association.	None.
Florida	**Indiana**	**Maryland**
Right of self organization plus required quarterly meetings between management and residents.	None.	None.
Michigan	**Minnesota**	**Missouri**
One resident as advisory member of board of directors.	None.	One resident as member of board of directors.

AAHA

None.

TABLE 11

ADVERTISING REGULATION

Arizona	California	Colorado
None.	If any third party is mentioned, must file a statement of financial responsibility with the state. Violation is a misdemeanor and can lead to revocation of certificate. Regulations require filing.	If any third party is mentioned, must include statement of its financial responsibility for the community. Violation is a misdemeanor.

Florida	Indiana	Maryland
Filing. If any third party is mentioned, must include statement of its financial responsibility for the community	A statement of financial responsibility by any affiliated charitable organization must be on file with the state.	Prohibited advertising must not be distributed; term not defined.

Michigan	Minnesota	Missouri
Filing. Agency can promulgate regulations on content.	None.	A statement of financial responsibility by any affiliated charitable organization must be on file with the state

AAHA

None.

TABLE 12

LIEN PROVISIONS AND PREFERRED CLAIMS

Arizona	California	Colorado
Lien as a precondition to certification. Subordinated to prior recorded encumbrances and permissive subordination to later recorded encumbrances.	Liens where necessary to secure performance of the continuing care contract. Subordinate to prior recorded liens.	Liens as a precondition to certification. Subordinated to prior recorded liens and permissive subordination to later recorded liens.

Florida	Indiana	Maryland
Perferred claim to residents on liquidation, but prior recorded liens retain their priority.	None.	None.

Michigan	Minnesota	Missouri
None.	Lien comes into existence when facility begins operation. No subordination at all.	None.

AAHA

None.

TABLE 13

RESPONSIBLE AGENCY

Arizona	California	Colorado
Department of insurance. No advisory council.	Department of Social Services. Eight member advisory board.	Department of Insurance. No advisory board.

Florida	Indiana	Maryland
Department of insurance. Seven member advisory council.	Department of Securities.	Office of Aging. No advisory board.

Michigan	Minnesota	Missouri
Corporation Securities Bureau of the Department of Commerce. No advisory board.	None.	Division of Insurance.

AAHA

Left to option of states. No advisory board.

TABLE 14

INVESTIGATIVE, ENFORCEMENT AND REHABILITATIVE POWERS

Arizona	California	Colorado
Examiners can conduct examinations as needed. Misdemeanor to violate. Rehabilitative authority	Inspections authorized at any time but annual audit can be relied on instead. Misdemeanor to violate. Rehabilitative authority.	Examinations when necessary. Injunctive relief. Misdemeanor to violate. Rehabilitative authority.

Florida	Indiana	Maryland
General examination authority. Injunctive relief. Felony and civil penalties for violations. Rehabilitative authority.	General investigative authority, plus subpoena power. Injunctive relief. Cease and desist orders allowed. Misdemeanor to violate. Rehabilitative authority.	General investigative authority. Injunctive relief. Misdemeanor to violate. Rehabilitative authority.

Michigan	Minnesota	Missouri
Limited power to investigate when records are missing, plus general investigative authority. Injunctive relief. Cease and desist power. Fines and imprisonment for violation.	Self-executing statute. Civil and criminal penalties for violation. Resident-initiated rehabilitation and liquidation procedures.	None.

AAHA

General investigative authority, plus subpoena power. Injunctive relief. Cease and desist orders allowed. No penalties for violation.

Chapter 4

Continuing Care Retirement Communities: Issues in Financial Management and Actuarial Prediction

Howard A. Winklevoss

In 1981, the Robert Wood Johnson Foundation and the Commonwealth Fund provided the University of Pennsylvania with $300,000 to conduct a study of the Continuing Care Retirement Community (CCRC) industry. The study had three purposes: to study the industry from empirical, actuarial, and legal views. Empirically, we wanted to find out what was out there, how many communities there were, what the physical configurations were, what the fee structures were, who sponsors them, and so forth. Therefore, we engaged in a massive empirical analysis. We identified about 300 or 400 communities that met our definition of a CCRC i.e., a community where, if you go into the medical center, you do not pay the per diem rate. In other words, a CCRC has an insurance element to the contract. There are another several hundred communities which are strictly fee for service types of communities which we did not classify as part of our study.

It is well known that many who conduct surveys are pleased to get a response rate of 30%. It is a tribute to the CCRC industry that we were able to get a response rate well over 75%, using a twenty page questionnaire. Thus, the industry was kind enough to cooperate and there now is a great deal of information which has been published in 2 volumes: (1) Winklevoss, Howard E., & Powell, Alwyn V. *Continuing Care Retirement Communities: An Empirical, Financial, and Legal Analysis.* Published for the Pension Research Council,

Howard E. Winklevoss, President, Winklevoss & Associates, Philadelphia, Pennsylvania; Adjunct Professor of Insurance, Wharton School, University of Pennsylvania.

Wharton School, University of Pennsylvania by Richard D. Irwin, Inc. Homewood, Ill. 1984. (2) *1982 Continuing Care Retirement Community Reference Directory* published by Human Services Research, Inc., Philadelphia.

The directory contains on a community by community basis fees and other features of CCRC's. It will be periodically updated by the American Association of Homes for the Aged.

A major aspect of the study was an actuarial analysis. One question asked was: is it possible to have a life care community with only 300 residents and, based on predictions of their life expectancies, financial projections and fee setting structures, to make the system work? The industry has been claiming for many years that it does not have the data, the information or the methodology to answer this question. Well, those excuses are no longer valid because our book sets forth all the ABC's of the actuarial end of the CCRC business in eight of its fourteen chapters. The final section of the book is on the existing regulations and more importantly, what the regulations should look like. Should regulation occur at the federal or state level? How detailed should it be? That section was written by Dave Cohen and a review of it appears in Chapter 3 of this volume. This material is very useful for the State of New York which may be considering what should be done, if anything, in regulating CCRC's.

One of the questions often asked is: are the current continuing care communities financially sound? We know that there are a small number of communities, such as Pacific Homes, which have gone bankrupt. But what about the rest of the communities? Because of our research conducted over the last two years, it is possible to answer that question though it was not easy to determine whether they are financially sound. Quite a large number of them seem to be financially sound and will continue to be financially sound. Through our study, and some consulting work done over the years, 15 communities were studied very intensely. Half of those communities were not financially sound, half of them were. That does not mean that half the communities out there are in trouble. The comparative method was used simply as an analytic tool. However, some communities that do ask a consultant for help are in trouble. But it seems that the industry as a whole is in good shape.

Returning to the question of whether or not the concept of life care for people in their mid-seventies can be made actuarially sound, that is difficult to answer because the industry is in its infancy. Quite a large number of communities will spring up over the next decade and there is a question of whether or not fees required to make the communities sound could only be affordable to the very wealthy. Our study indicates that the entry fees and the monthly fees charged by a large number of communities are just about right; in other words, an entry fee on the order of forty, fifty or sixty thousand dollars and a monthly fee ranging from $700 to $1000 depending on such factors as the degree of continuous health care, the construction costs and so forth, is realistic. It is estimated that between 15% and 25% of the people in the over age 75 category could easily afford a CCRC, taking into account their home ownership. And it might even be as high as 1/3 of this age group. It is probably not as high as 1/2 and it may never be as high as 2/3 of all the aged people who could afford to fund this type of care.

However, if there are funds coming from the community at large or other organizations to subsidize them then more will be able to afford it. However, it should be noted that 20% of the people over the age 75 represent quite a large number relative to the 50,000 people that the industry is now serving.

A major problem in the financial management of a life care community is the very deceptive nature of the income and cash flow of these communities over the first decade and a half of their existence. When you open up a community, you get a tremendous influx of funds in the form of entry fees, while the health care utilization of the residents admitted does not accelerate for about 10 or 15 years. What that means is that the overseers of that community have to have enough patience and fortitude to reserve the monies that they are receiving during the first 10 years until there is an inevitable increase in health care utilization. Lack of reserves has been a big problem. As was noted above, when communities start out they have quite a bit of money, health care utilization is low, and they run the finances of the community in such a way that the amount of money coming in equals the amount going out. Thus, a substantial hidden liability begins to build up. Then if they should have a minor adverse experience, such as a cash flow problem, they find out that there is a tremendous unfunded health care liability, which is very difficult to remedy financially.

A number of factors contribute to lack of reserves. First, generally accepted accounting principles (GAAP) are not adequate for the management of these communities if they are going to set fees to reserve for the long term health care obligation. This does not imply that GAAP should not be used; certainly they should but they are not adequate when running a "mini-insurance company." This has already been recognized by both the pension and the insurance industries. Second, life care communities do not often have boards which have a lot of time to spend on finance issues and often they do not understand the true nature of the financial commitment of a CCRC. Moreover, they tend to be offended if in the early years revenues exceed expenses. As soon as this happens the board feels that it does not need to increase fees or suggests only a modest increase because it looks like the community is making a profit, and the last thing board members want to do is profit from the people they are trying to serve. Generally, GAAP accounting statements will show substantial profits every year during the first 10 years if the fees are correct. However they are not really profits; they are funds that are going to be needed to support the health care obligation later on. But the combination of the deceptive nature of GAAP accounting, the non-profit aspect of the homes, and the lack of understanding that the health care guarantee is a deferred obligation which should be funded, causes communities to underprice themselves. If they are lucky enough to get through the first 15 years, then the chances are good that they can continue with revenues equaling expenditures, because everything will have reached a fairly steady state. Unfortunately in the last years, inflation has caused a lot of communities to be unable to get through the maturation period, and they have run into trouble. Third, another accounting factor which is problematic is the earning of entry fees which is done uniformly wrong across the industry. When you receive a $50,000 entry fee, it is important for the board to set up the right mechanism by which that entry fee can be considered income to the community. If one considers that the entry fee is to be income in the first year, one is going to lose money every year thereafter. How can one assume that the $50,000 entry fee is earned over the lifetime of the individual? Half of the communities earn it over the life expectancy of the individual. If a person is going to live 15 years, they will receive their income stream at the rate of 1/15 of the $50,000 per year. Half the people are going to live beyond the life expectancy, a period during which their care will be more expensive. So if you earn all of the money up until a person's life expectancy, obviously you have earned that money too fast. The group of communities surviving out there are the ones which have recognized that this is a problem. They earn the entry fee over a longer period than life expectancy. However, when they do this, they must recognize that they violate the fundamental principle of management accounting which dictates that your revenues should match your expenses and that when you have an expense stream that will escalate because of increased health care utilization, you can avoid having monthly fees increased by more than inflation only by earning a very small portion of the entry fee initially and then by gradually increasing the amount. To date, no communities seem to be earning entry fees correctly. Thus, they are all in the unfortunate position of earning what looks like a profit. Since boards of directors do not want to make a profit, they do not pass proper fee increases on to residents and they start creating an unfunded health care liability.

It is not true that you cannot predict the future health care utilization of 300 residents. Most people belong to a pension plan and the pension industry faces the same problem. When an employer hires an employee at age 30, he/she has to determine how long that person will stay with the firm, whether or not he will die, at what age he will die, whether or not he will become disabled and whether or not he will stay in employment to retirement to start collecting on a pension plan about 35 years from day of employment. The pension industry asks: when an employee does collect, how long is he/she going to live beyond say the year 2000 to receive that pension? Obviously it is not possible for an actuary to estimate this for an employer with 300 employees with 100% confidence. But pension plans—and there are hundreds of thousands of pension plans in this country—go through the calculations to see how much reserve money they should have and how much they should put into the plan during one year to head towards a moving target. The moving target is the true liability because it is never really known.

The same actuarial principles apply to CCRC's. It is impossible to predict the liability for each new resident entering a community or what the liability is for the entire community with 100% accuracy, but it is possible to approach such a prediction and it can be tracked over time. The insurance aspect of CCRC's is no different from that of pension plans, life insurance companies, or health insurance companies. There are good actuarial scientific principles that should help any actuary sit down with these communities so that they can maintain their financial well being over time.

One of the unique features about a CCRC is that it is a multi-million dollar operation. Although a community budget each year might be $2,000,000 to $5,000,000, few seem to hire an actuary or an accountant to do some financial planning. It is difficult to under-

stand this reluctance. In point of fact the cost of hiring such personnel is not very great. If every CCRC in the country did an actuarial
valuation, the revenue would be something on the order of
$5,000,000 to the actuarial community. The revenue to the actuarial
community on behalf of pension plans alone is well in excess of
$500,000,000. In fact, if there is any problem, it would be that it is
difficult to get the actuarial community interested enough to serve
the industry. If these communities are going to work, they have to
be run like businesses and that means: one, hire professional
marketing people especially when a community is developed in a
new location. Two, hire accountants, lawyers, actuaries and so
forth. If you do not want to make those kinds of expenditures, do not
get involved with a CCRC. All the good intentions in the world in
caring for the aged will not keep these organizations financially
sound without professional management expertise.

With regard to regulation, those of us involved in the study were
going to write model legislation, but we were talked out of it for a
good reason. We do not know enough about the industry. What one
might develop as model legislation might be perfect for the one
community used as a model, but it would not be perfect for another
state or another type of community. Our final recommendation was
that legislation should not be written at the federal level; it should be
written at the state level because experimentation in legislation is
needed. Dave Cohen has done an admirable job listing all the areas
he thinks could be regulated and why, with regard to the financial or
actuary reserve issue. There are regulations for pensions and there
are regulations for insurance companies and continuing care communities have elements of both. It is too soon to propose detailed
regulations about what the financial reserve should be. But minimal-
ly regulations might say that CCRCs need to have a certified public
accountant certify that their financial statements are correct and also
that there should be a certified actuarial review.

A couple of weeks ago Senator Heinz asked me to take a look at a
prospectus on a community that recently went bankrupt. Although
he is a Harvard graduate, he studied the prospectus the night before
and said, "You know, I cannot tell whether this is a good investment or not, what am I missing?" I put him at ease by saying that no
one, no matter how knowledgeable could assess from a feasibility
study whether or not that community was going to make it. The
types of forecasts that have been done in feasibility studies are em-
barrassing, sloppy, and too short. In a five-year forecast on a life

care community, nothing can go wrong if you can sell to full occupancy; if you cannot get full occupancy all the actuarial analyses are not going to help you. That is why marketing is so important. Most of the feasibility studies are done by deterministic methodology which assumes that a fraction of people will die each year. In the book that reports our study we describe a procedure where, when you have 300 people, there is a possible range of deviations. If not enough people die, you do not have the apartment turnover expected and thus no new corresponding entry fees. A methodology that deals with this problem is mentioned in the book.

There is a major need for a national data base providing accurate information on how long people live in CCRCs. Our studies show that life expectancies among residents are 20% longer than those of the general population. We do not know why. It is not clear whether this is because CCRCs only admit people who are healthy or because easy access to health care mantains their health. This is an area for future research. A very curious finding occurred in communities where residents had completely free access to health care with no additional cost as compared to those communities that required residents to pay an additional fee for health care: the health care utilization was lower. That is, where there was free access to health care it was used less, we are not quite sure why. It is quite possible that there is a connection between the feeling of relief at having health care readily available and good physical health. Future research needs to be done in these areas.

In conclusion it should be stressed that there is a need for data to be developed so that communities can share information. The insurance industry has been building such a data base for many years. Prudential, Metropolitan, Equitable, and other companies meet each year and share their experiences. Together they develop national mortality tables which everybody uses. The CCRC industry should do the same.

Chapter 5

Ethical Issues in Continuing Care

Monsignor Charles J. Fahey

It is important to clarify the values underlying decisions concerning what activity we wish to encourage or discourage and allow or disallow through government action. It is particularly important to do so at this time of increased need and of constrained resources.

Values dictate individual and group behavior. Public policy emanates from personal values articulated in the political process. Our pluralism can make it difficult to come to a concensus on which values should be expressed in statutes, regulation or reimbursement policies. The process becomes even more complex and confounded completely at times because of differing perspectives of persons with the same values as to the prudential course to follow in a given situation. Yet the identification of those values which are to be considered is not merely an academic exercise but is at the heart of policy debate.

While perspectives from economics, political science, sociology and even psychology are introduced to public decision making, the ethics of public acts is rarely identified explicitly through value implications of policy decisions. They are there to be discovered.

The several states view their roles differently in the area of continuing care. Some merely prescind from the specific area and depend on generic statutes of regulations to control behavior in this area. Others such as California, have evolved rather detailed statutes which are designed specifically to deal with continuing care. New York has chosen a policy which virtually precludes development of such programs.

We are examining New York's policy approach specifically and it is my task to contribute an ethical framework and some "value insights" which ought to be part of the deliberations as we consider

---

Msgr. Fahey is Director, Third Age Center, Fordham University, New York City.

65

whether New York State should continue or modify its current approach.

There is nothing mysterious about ethics. It speaks of the "oughtness" of things. It attempts to identify that which corresponds to the dignity of human beings. It struggles with such concepts as beauty, truth, goodness and justice; abstractions yes, but the very staff of human enterprise.

We should note that while ethics and morality are closely associated, they are distinguishable. Morality speaks to the "oughtness" of human acts but it is dependent largely on insights from a religious tradition. On the other hand, ethics is dependent on insights of "unaided reason." In practice each is influenced by the other since they address the values of the same human experience within the same cultural milieu.

At the heart of the ethical reflection is applying insights from all disciplines to a given act and synthesizing them into a logical whole. The process is faulty to the degree that a perspective, whether historical or current, remains outside the analysis and synthesis.

Public policy grows out of personal and group "values" as mediated by the political process. A policy, a product of compromise as it always is, takes on a value or ethical perspective of its own.

In the inquiry under consideration in this volume, there are at least three principle actors with a stake in the public policy question: the potential user of the service, the provider and society as a whole. The legimate interests of each must be considered.

THE USER

The life care community offers a prospective client a place to live supported by various services including specialized nursing care for a one time substantial fee plus a periodic (usually monthly) service charge. The purchaser may establish an equity interest in the facility or merely be entitled to "life tenancy."

The number of such facilities coupled with projections of dramatic growth are evidence that some persons find this arrangement to be desirable. While many facilities have attractive amenities including well designed physical plants, meals and stimulating intellectual environments, the principle attraction for most persons is "security." Such places offer clients the assurance that possible future dependency needs will be met. It offers the individual or couple the opportunity to provide for themselves while they are still "in control."

Ironically the same elements which afford security may have deleterious effects upon the individual. Taking up residence in such a community involves a significant commitment. While persons of different levels of affluence will invest differing proportions of their resources in the arrangement, the very nature of such communities demands rather substantial outlays of financial resources, as well as time and interest on the part of those who utilize them.

Such aspects as the requirement that persons participate in a meal program tend to create an institutional approach to living. For one person this is an important element in security and community, for another it creates dependency. For some it will offer new stimulation, for others it may further a process of withdrawal.

From the perspective of an individual, such an arrangement seems to be a reasonable option to meet one's present and future needs. The structure does not, in and of itself, preclude a person from being a complete human being.

PROVIDER OF SERVICES

As in every exchange of goods and services, there are responsibilities, on the part of the seller and the buyer. However, in this instance, special responsibilities arise from the duration of the relationship, the vulnerability of the buyer, and the complexity of the services to be provided.

The seller must state accurately that which he will and will not do as well as delineate the processes which will be used if there is a change in the buyer's health status.

Among these issues, which both the seller and the regulator must consider, is the ability of any seller, no matter how much good will there is, to provide long range assurances in circumstances involving so many variables.

While the basic framework of the relationship is delineated in an original agreement, the relationship between the parties tends to be somewhat fluid. Projections in the area of longevity have proven to be inaccurate over the years. It is difficult to predict the future needs of an individual. Furthermore, the potential for conflict between the individual and the seller in terms of how needs are to be met is real. In some instances, they will not perceive "need" in the same way.

The factors motivating the parties in meeting commonly perceived need may be quite different leading to different courses of action. Thus, there is the necessity of an agreed upon process to adjudicate disputes which should be part of the original agreement.

Increased longevity and the concomitant likelihood of disability (including a greater likelihood of some intellectual deficit) can give rise to management difficulties since a seller has assumed a responsibility for the well-being of a potentially frail person.

The difficulty of meeting need and expectancy is complicated further by the limitations on the seller's control of resources which might be appropriate in a given situation; as needs become more complex, so too do means of meeting them. The field of aging is no exception. Rarely will a provider or seller be able to "control" and "deliver" the full complex of desirable and/or needed services despite a commitment to do so.

It is important to note the inherent though probably not insurmountable conflict between the purchaser's desire for security and the provider's need to provide a conservative program for meeting need.

Such a conflict can also be perceived within the provider organization. those who do marketing have a strong motivation to "sell" security in terms of the comprehensive program while those faced with long term management responsibilities likely will counsel a conservative approach. It is essential such issues be resolved "before the fact" within this type of organization.

Even a cursory explanation of continuing care in our country reveals dramatic and indeed tragic examples of poor planning and unethical practices as providers have failed to resolve these issues.

SOCIETY IN GENERAL

There is a consensus in American public life that individuals should be free to act if others are not injured. On the other hand, there is a concensus that government has the responsibility to enter into the exchange of goods and services in those instances where the buyer may be vulnerable to exploitation. Policy makers find themselves faced with two broadly held concepts which may be in conflict.

Since New York is so singular in its approach, clearly there is a need to reexamine the values which dictate its current approach in the face of a need for new resources for meeting needs.

New York's stringent approach grows from the State's general, long held social policy perspective. New York has had a deep concern for vulnerable people and has responded quickly to abuse. Some might observe that New York tends to over-respond. Unfortunately, we have examples of poor planning if not out and out fraud in New York State. However, are there new factors which may lead New York to a different policy?

One reality is that there is a general acceptance of continuing care by states outside New York. Another reality is the increased popularity of this program. Some New Yorkers seek this type of program out of the state. Another consideration is the improvement in the actuarial art and its application to this field specifically. And we now have additional experience with the regulatory approach of other states.

CONCLUSIONS

There is a need to develop social structures which offer incentives to older persons to spend resources on themselves. It is desirable that they utilize goods and services which will enrich their lives. Apparently, in many states continuing care communities offer such enrichment.

Still questions persist. Has the state of the art developed sufficiently to assure the prudent buyer and seller that projections can be made concerning future needs? Unlike general insurance programs, changes in need and costs can not be dealt with by selling new policies or by changing premiums (unless such changes are provided for in an original agreement).

Were this approach to become popular in New York, how would it effect the certificate of need process? Would it lead to two levels of care, one for the affluent another for the poor? How would use of such facilities affect an individual's eligibility for Medicaid? Should such programs develop "dedicated nursing homes," i.e., exclusively for their own constituency? Could such dedicated facilities sustain themselves? How would they interact with community systems of care?

Were the approach to be liberalized at the state level, potential providers as well as users would still need to resolve the sorts of questions listed above.

PART III:
EVOLVING MANAGEMENT STRUCTURES:
A CASE STUDY

Introduction to Part III

In *Chapter 6,* Frank Elliott and Stephanie Elliott, founders of the Continuing Care Retirement Village at Pine Run, Doylestown, Pennsylvania trace the development of this CCRC prototype from an organizational perspective. Their detailed descriptions of various management structures provide a practical insight into the problems and functioning of such a complex organization. They are careful to point out that in spite of a great deal of experimentation and risk-taking during the years since its inception, Pine Run today is a well-run facility where residents together with the professional staff are involved in all phases of the community's organization and management.

Chapter 6

Evolving Management Structures: A Case Study of a Life Care Village at Pine Run, Doylestown, Bucks County, Pennsylvania

Frank E. Elliott
Stephanie H. Elliott

This paper attempts to delineate the journey of one continuing care retirement community—Pine Run Community (PRC) of Doylestown, Pennsylvania—through the cycle of differing management structures that were found useful while passing from the initial opening of the community and the move-in of its first residents to the present ongoing operation. It is believed that persons initiating such a community might find it of value to hear a predecessor's experiences in structuring the management of this rather complex, always surprising, entity.

Continuing care retirement communities (CCRCs) can be Protean creatures to manage. They may be at one moment a resort hotel, at another a social support network and always must be simply "home" for the elders living there. Staff can range from health care professionals to high school age waitresses who must become "professional" gerontologists to do their jobs well. Park facilities, sidewalks, roads and grounds must be reminiscent of an English estate, while being elder-safe even in the most violent weather. Depending on the extent of service guarantees, expert long range financial analysis and forecasting becomes crucial.

Always, there is a unique need to focus on the individual, which begins at PRC with the method of setting fees and an extensive set of service guarantees described below. PRC's concept of aging infuses the entire evolution of its management structure which is the main subject for discussion in this paper.

Pine Run Community is a privately sponsored life care village operating in Doylestown, Pennsylvania, since 1976. An unusual group of older Americans bring to the community a new way of life at an advanced age that they have themselves helped to design and regulate, and which they helped to prescribe.

Pine Run members come from all over America and Europe. Some of the members have followed their children here who hold good positions in nearby metropolitan areas. A few members have returned to the source of their roots and upbringing. The majority, outliving friends and family, have come in search of social continuity, secured independence and decent comprehensive medical support when needed. Many members of the community joined when they were "ready"; that is, having planned ahead, the day arrived when the house became too much to handle or support was, or soon would be, needed in caring for a loved one.

Presently, Pine Run encompasses a population of 500 members and patients whose average age is 81 years. The community will *always* remain predominately female (70%). Couples represent nearly 60% of the population. The majority of the members have advanced education, are well traveled and maintain long standing relations in church and club. The majority also, especially the women, maintain good health, stay involved with good nutrition and make repeated use of the available social and medical supports, home health care and diagnostic services. Over 85% of the members monitor themselves by checking in with the medical staff at least once a month. 60% of the members still drive automobiles; a few of the drivers are in their low nineties. Several members remain active in their professions or businesses. A significant majority (over 80%) participate in volunteer efforts at Pine Run and in the broader community.

The major complaints of old age in the community naturally reflect the predominance of women: arterial hypertension, pain in locomotion, poor eyesight and general anxiety arising from diminishing of accustomed psycho-physiological performance.

Outwardly, PRC nestles in resort-like ambiance on a 41-acre tract abutting a lake and wildlife area. Facilities include 300 terraced apartments clustered as 19 "neighborhoods" more or less equidistant from a 24,000 foot social service, recreation and shopping mall center called "the hub." Completing the site are a six-mile circulation network of paths, covered sidewalks and roadways; and a five-story, 236 bed geriatric rehabilitation "medical hotel" which climbs grade a step at a time allowing direct access to an outdoor pavilion for each floor. More than 250 full time equivalent employees (350 personnel) work around the clock, seven days a week, serving community members and patients annually. Indeed, PRC is a self-sufficient health care town having its own utility, fire and emergency alert systems, voting district, hospital, shopping mall, inns, streets and covered walkways, "town hall" and administration offices.

Inwardly, PRC is a thoughtfully planned integrated network of life support, nurture and leisure systems that have been rigorously set in place to satisfy two geriatric scales—a scale of adaptable physical plant and a scale of multidisciplinary service options. These enable community life to keep reappearing in new forms for the individuals who live here. The community and its buildings experience constant redesign and readaptation to meet the needs of the changing older body, and management programs are constantly redefined to meet changing mobility and self support limitations.

PINE RUN COMMUNITY AS ONE CCRC PROTOTYPE

Pine Run is a CCRC that offers extensive—indeed, maximum—health care guarantees, providing almost all medical services, physician and nursing care, rehabilitation services, custodial care and prescription drugs, up to the end of life, as well as standard housekeeping, maintenance, meals, recreation, transportation, etc.[1] It is not the client who must adapt to the organization, but the organization which must understand in depth and adapt to the client if these extensive guarantees are to be met. And as will be described below, financial forecasting takes on crucial importance.

Fees

Traditionally residents of CCRC's (called members) pay a fixed entry fee and a monthly rate that can change within limits. Such fees are usually an across-the-board schedule related primarily to the size of apartment the member will occupy. Within market possibilities for pricing, age and gender information on CCRC members supply a generalized basis for the fee schedule and for periodic financial analyses and forecasts.[2] By contrast Pine Run has pioneered in individually tailoring each entering member's fees to his own unique financial, age, gender, health and biographic characteristics, focusing management from the outset on in-depth actuarially-based understanding of each client as an individual.[3]

Service Guarantees

Residents in CCRCs do not own their apartments. Rather, the membership fees purchase a bundle of services guaranteed in an individual contract between each member and the community. Such guarantees vary widely today in different communities. Some communities offer extensive guarantees; in others, they are very limited. It is not unusual currently for a CCRC to guarantee little more than is covered by Medicare, e.g., perhaps 180 days of custodial nursing at the member's previous monthly rate, after which he will pay fee-for-service.[4]

Levels of Care

PRC management also must meet the challenge of offering a number of levels of care as part of its continuing care spectrum. Beyond the basic apartment program for active and healthy elders, PRC has a diagnostic and out-patient center and several levels of home health care. Offered in the Medical Center are "medical hotel" services, personal care and intermediate, skilled, ambulatory confused and long-term custodial programs, each sub-defined into several sublevels.

Private Family Ownership

Pine Run and its related entities are a family-owned corporation. Being in private ownership, Pine Run cannot look to charitable fund-raising to assist with management problems, and its management structures have been affected by that fact.

Whatever the ownership base, however, the challenge to management is always to be as creative as possible in the effort to do as much as possible with the resources available. The comments below are offered in the hope that they may have stimulating aspects for any management, whether privately owned or charitably based.

Member-Inclusive Management Structures Reflect a Recognition of Aging as Dynamic

PRC management structures described in this paper reveal not only the above-noted effort to *understand* the organization's aged members, but also an effort actually to *integrate* the members into the management structures. This is based on the belief and experience that aging is not entirely a decline. The biological growth curve of an individual may peak at mid-twenty and then decline.[5,6,7] Social life and skills may plateau at or after midlife, only to decline in late life in face of physical and mental losses and society's ineptness at providing either roles or support to those of advanced age.[8-12] At PRC, however, a cultural/adaptational curve is observed that is more often an upward dynamic than a decline.[13-17] (See Figure 1.)

Again and again, at PRC one sees elders who are continuously recreating a sense of normal life in an active, engaging and productive way in the face of ever-worsening chronic physical and mental problems, thus continuously developing and strengthening their personhood to handle the next challenge in daily survivorship. Negative curves notwithstanding, residents maintain their own proper schedule of aging with a positive attitude. This phenomenon is termed the "cultural/adaptational curve" at PRC.

Recognizing this growth and strength in its members, PRC (or any CCRC) can become a microcosm where management has a unique opportunity to study in depth, through the practical actions of its members, the ways in which self-reliant and independent living can be sustained in advanced age. The residents are the experts in what is needed and wanted. They often hold the best answers as to how these needs can efficiently and satisfactorily be delivered. Thus, at PRC, management structures are sought that allow the member to be trainer and leader in the management process. In the management evolution described below, there is a continuing effort to encourage such a development.

The "Village-Effect" in Management Structure

Pine Run Community, like many CCRCs, breathes, lives, works and expects as a village. Executives, employees and members are drawn by a complex information-sharing network into one social body. The management structure of such an entity, to be most effec-

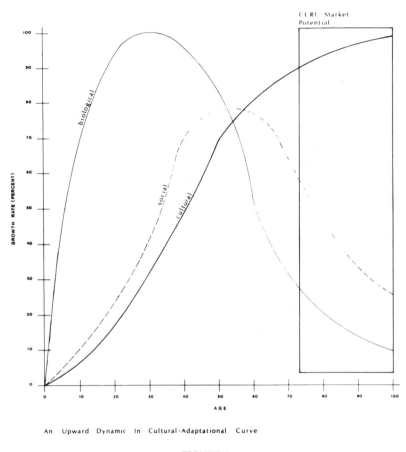

An   Upward   Dynamic   In   Cultural-Adaptational   Curve

FIGURE 1

tive, must be harmonious with this fact. The search for this harmony
also is clear in the growth from structure to structure described
below.

EVOLVING FORMS OF PRC MANAGEMENT STRUCTURE

Organizational forms at Pine Run have developed with the evolving life cycle of the community itself. Management's aim was to put
in place the most appropriate form of organization for the upcoming
phase of critical growth that it would be experiencing.[18] These
phases were: (1) coordinating client move-in during the transition

from construction to start-up operations; (2) grounding the new organization; (3) operating as an experienced "going concern."

Pre-Opening Member Involvement

An effort to tap the experts—the aged members themselves—has characterized PRC's entire management experience. Thus, even before the Community opened, when barely half the buildings were roughed in, two workshop days were held at six-month intervals on the construction site. At each session, approximately 150 members-to-be from all states in New England and the Middle Atlantic region, and from farther south and west as well, traveled to Doylestown to voice their opinions about the plans for facilities, decor, management policy and self-governance. Issues decided ranged from "shall there be a cocktail lounge" to member election of a committee from among themselves to formulate a constitution and member organization ready to coordinate with management on opening day.

I. The Initial Management Structure: The Traditional, Multi-Tier Hierarchy (1976-1977)

Pine Run opened in June, 1976. For the first few years, members were moving in and both members and managers were becoming adjusted to life as a community. In this initial period the traditional, multi-tiered, hierarchical form of management structure shown in Exhibit 1 was used, some form of which is typical of most American social service organizations.

In government or human service organizations, as distinct from business, this hierarcical organization is frequently held together by some individual with expertise central to the service being performed, often characterized as such by licensure, e.g., the psychiatrist head of a state department of mental health, the licensed nursing home administrator, the minister heading a church home. (For PRC the central figure was an individual experienced in non-profit sponsored life care who served as Community Director.) Services are then substructured under this central control. While one would say they are organized by task, e.g., food service, maintenance, etc., they are in fact often grouped and shaped by the crises that arise out of countervailing pressures and demands by board policymakers, management and clients. The structure, therefore, as it evolves, is

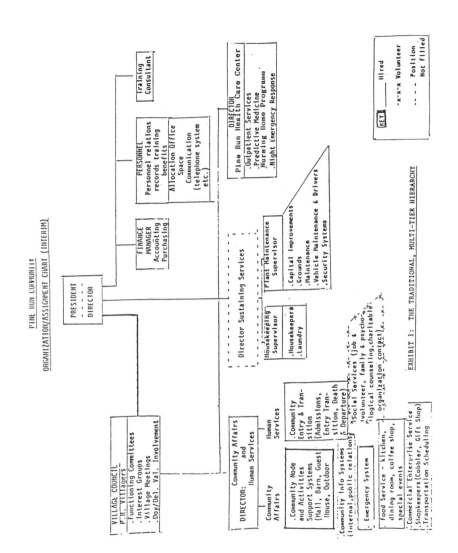

EXHIBIT 1: THE TRADITIONAL, MULTI-TIER HIERARCHY

often deputized in a random, intuitive fashion rather than in the rational, analytic manner often experienced, for example, in the field of manufacturing.

One readily sees this pattern reflected at PRC in Exhibit 1 where, for example, the Director of Community Afairs and Human Services had responsibility for Food Service but not Housekeeping; for the Emergency Alert System which involved Health Center personnel but not for the Health Center itself; for transportation scheduling but not vehicle maintenance and drivers—clearly a mixed bag.

For all its imbalances, however, this hierarchical structure served three important purposes as PRC phased members into residence, and management into experience/expertise.

1. Crises Management Without Cross-Training

People moving into the community needed quick, "hands on," person-to-person management service because of the crisis of continued construction (noise, dirt, strangers). Furthermore, the multidisciplinary nature of continuing care meant that PRC would ultimately be cross-training its personnel to perform each other's jobs, an effort which had not yet had time to develop. Altogether, a structure that related supervision to type of crisis served well.

2. A Familiar Order

The one-boss hierarchy is a structure with which people are familiar. For PRC elders, it was apt to be the only structure they had ever seen in operation. It gave at least the appearance of order and stability, in a disorderly period, helping to stabilize the community's effort to become one social body.

3. Ease of Initiating Member Involvement

Finally, again because traditional hierarchy was a structure that members readily understood, it was easy to begin to build member input into PRC's organizational style. The Villager government, begun at the pre-opening workshops, had early established its own structure and constitution. Hand-in-hand function with management was developed. Villager Committees were created to advise each component of management—grounds, food service, marketing, health care, entry fee investment, financial reporting and status, etc.

The Villager President and Vice President met weekly with the Community Director and Associate Director to create a commonly agreed upon strategy for solving intractable problems—a strategy that often involved some actions by staff and others by members or member groups. Management and members thus co-sponsored the development of a strong Villager member organization, and ultimately a patients' council, able to give input to each aspect of management's activity.

II. Learning the Business In Depth: The Technobureaucratic, "Conglomerate" Structure (1978-1981)

During move-in, a sense of community had been built that included both staff and members. Avenues for member input to management had been opened. Simultaneously, from 1975 through 1976, with both the Winklevoss firm (see Chapter 4) and with the accounting firm of Peat, Marwick and Mitchell, PRC had been pioneering methods for actuarial forecasting related to "life care" guarantees. This work continued with the help of a medically trained PRC staff mathematician. The resulting forecasts told PRC the same story of future shortfalls that such forecasts told many other CCRC's a year or two later when the whole industry began to investigate such methods.

By 1977 PRC found itself facing these newly-discovered long-term management exigencies, and also a number of more immediate organizational demands:

1. Cost Control

PRC needed better day-to-day financial controls in order to maximize the service it was giving for the available dollar. Continuing care involves a great variety of services exposed to change, while relying on a relatively fixed revenue stream. Thus, there is a continuing problem of watchdogging unnecessary costs, while expanding necessary ones. At PRC this is called "watching the little things."

2. Routinized Forecasting

As a CCRC providing maximum service guarantees, PRC needed to routinize the receipt and processing of sufficient data from all parts of its operations to allow very accurate, repeatable, 5-to-15 year forecasts of service needs and costs, a move to minimize long-term financial surprises.

3. Building a Foundation Based on the Computer

It seemed both these needs could best be met in the 1980s by a comprehensive, interfacing computer operation which *would have* to be developed as soon as possible (1979-1981).

4. Diversification for Added Revenues

The management of PRC felt it might find a solution to overall long-term financial security for the Community by diversifying its operations into related but independent revenue-producing subsidiaries through a long-term borrowing strategy. The idea was that after becoming expert through their work at PRC, company subentities might expand to sell their services to other organizations or "life care communities," creating profits that would bring added cash "into the till" from sources other than PRC members.

5. Training

Finally, there was a training need. PRC management wanted each person who worked in the Community to become a gerontological expert, knowledgeable about aging and the aged person's needs, while also becoming a professional in the task assigned. In fact, because of the holistic nature of the member's demand for service and support, PRC has found that it needs a new kind of professional, not only gerontologically sensitive and task-knowledgeable, but also a "jack of all trades" when emergency need arises.

In an attempt to meet this new set of challenges, PRC experimented for serveral years with a management structure similar to that of a multi-national conglomerate.[20] As may be seen in the chart in Exhibit 2, PRC structured its small social service organization into a number of separate "companies." People involved in non-medical operating management became Life Care Management, Inc., centermost in the chart. Medical aspects became a separate entity already serving outsiders, the Pine Run Health Care Center, Inc., shown on the right leg of the chart. Food Service for both operations was organized as a Division (chart, lower corner) with potential for catering beyond Pine Run. Maintenance, laundry and

EXHIBIT 2: THE TECHNOBUREACRATIC "CONGLOMERATE" STRUCTURE

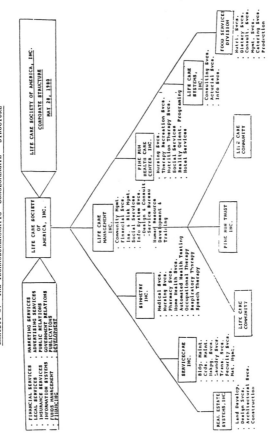

84

housekeeping activities similarly became Service Care, Inc. while Life Care Society of America, Inc. became a holding company of topmost management.

How could forming such a highly rationalized, pyramidical conglomerate structure with only 350 employees help solve the financial and training challenges PRC was facing?

First, the comprehensive financial and behavioral data desired for control and forecasting purposes at a level then unique in the life care field would require several years of effort, introduction of a powerful computer and an initial oversized high-level professionalism in staffing. The conglomerate structure allowed us to attract such staff even though they would not be needed at PRC itself over the long pull. Secondly, the conglomerate structure would give a detailed organizational scaffolding by which to collect and on which to hang buckets of data. Finally, subsidiary activity by the extra, high level staff might enable them to pay for themselves and thus remain at PRC.

For the first two purposes, the experiment proved highly successful. Less successful was the third—the attempt to provide additional *long-term* income to PRC and retain long-term high level staffing through subsidiary activities. National and regional economic difficulties that had commenced in 1974 and continued throughout the decade largely aborted this strategy. Thus, once PRC was computer-based, Phase II came to an end. The scaffolding of the conglomerate structure was dismantled and the highly professional but expensive top level of management went their separate ways.

PRC then made a hoped for discovery. A subgroup of experts had been developing at lower levels of management within the subsidiaries. These "comers" within the staff knew policy and procedure by heart. They had often written it. They had been trained in depth and across-the-board in their respective subsidiary areas. They had been in close contact with PRC members while solving problems in those areas. They were, in short, professionals at "the PRC way" of handling their specialty—whether food service, social service, security, etc. In addition, management training and special courses on aging had been developed for their benefit. They had become gerontologically wise through both formalized training and experience. Lastly, they had been the ones responsible on a day-to-day basis for setting up the terminal-to-computer relay stations throughout the community that reported member, program and service data for centralized analyses and reports. These "comers" were ready to form the core of the third phase in PRC's management journey described below.

III. Structuring the Ongoing Operation: A Team-Based, Computer-Informed Synergy (1981. . .)[19,21,22]

We come now to the current day. Resting as PRC does now on the computer-based financial control and forecasting abilities just described, PRC now is continuing an effort to further embody in its management structure both the sense of Pine Run as one social body (the "village effect" referred to earlier), and the related fuller integration of the members into management.

The current structure which is still developing is essentially a team management system where members are part of the team, and where the computer acts as technical executive. Elements, illustrated in the chart labeled Exhibit 3, include:

1. *The Core Team* of five management leaders who operate together as Top Boss (top of chart).

2. *Villager Participation* through the Villager Board, the Villager Executive Committee, the Villager Liaison Committee (top of chart), and through a series of Villager subcommittees shown in the chart as boxed "VMC"'s attached to each management program.

3. *The Team Assembly* by which the work of the Community is organized as a series of thirty gerontologically attuned service programs whose leaders meet regularly both as a group, and also individually with the assigned Villager subcommittee.

4. *The Computer as Technical Executive* represented first in Exhibit 3 as a series of computer terminal ideographs attached to each team assembly program, and secondly as the computer information system complex and its related Management Systems staff at the bottom of the chart.

The Core Team as Top Boss

The Core Team meets weekly and acts jointly as "CEO." At the same time, each member of the team directs one of the major service domains purposely designed with overlapping program responsibilities:

Hospitality: marketing and admissions, member social services, quality assurance, recreation assistance to members (who, however,

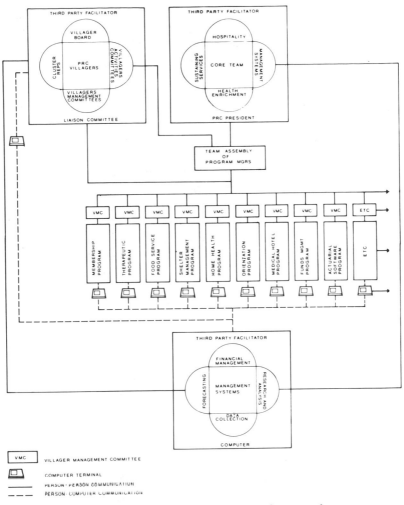

Exhibit 3: A Team-Based, Computer-Informed, Single Tier Organization Structure

prefer to retain full control of plans for this area) and multiple milieu and psychotherapies.

Health Enrichment: medical, geriatric, diagnostic and home health services.

Sustaining Services: nutrition, maintenance, grounds, laundry, housekeeping, security, transportation and special events.

Management Systems: funds management, financial reporting and forecasting, information systems, geriatric and behavioral analysis.

PRC President: long-term policy development and ex-officio third party mediator between and among managers, members and patients.

Why use a core team as top boss, rather than the traditional single, "CEO" head of the hierarchy?

PRC's first aim is to generate maximum effectiveness in setting social and medical support priorities. In a human service operation there is never enough of any resource to do all the things one wants to do. Priorities have to be set among organizational areas regarding the timing of projects and equitable sharing of available capital, material and employee and member manpower and expertise. At PRC, the Core Team decides together on these priorities. It is their experience that when all get behind the final decision and all can explain to members and on-line staff why some projects must be delayed, then one seldom hears that retreat from responsibility: "I don't know—the boss said so."

All organizations experience conflicts where responsibility overlaps and where gray areas in policy-making occur. This is especially true in human service organizations. PRC decided to bring the problem right to the surface by purposely overlapping jurisdictions, e.g., having some medical center therapies run by the hospitality Core Team Leader (see Core Team domains described above). In this way, the Core Team structure enables the interfaced resolution of those surfaced conflicts. Team members, perforce, recognize their interdependent relationship. They encourage and demand of each other harmonious conflict resolution, thereby maximizing a community-wide sense of common purpose and harmony.

The essence of human services management is responsiveness, especially in emergencies. PRC finds that with team management, the various branches of the organization are accustomed to working closely together, know each other's day-to-day problems, and can more readily make decisions "on their feet" in an emergency or fill in for each other when needed.

Because each team member is responsible not only for creating and meeting his own program area's business plan, but also for negotiating with the others the company's final master business plan, PRC finds that day-to-day financial performance in each area stays more closely attuned to overall, agreed upon management and membership goals.

Villagers were at first concerned to have no single "top boss" to whom to take complaints and concerns. They are finding now, that with no "absolute monarch," they have much greater access to the decision-making process, and greater likelihood of being able to work their will. There are more avenues of approach, more possibilities of repeating an approach, and persuasive possibilities are maximized.

The Member As Team Participant[21]

Members at Pine Run, as described earlier, are formally structured into the management organization. More than a matter of business goodwill, this decision by management to have members "privy" to the inner workings of the business is based upon a definite deference given to the long-living member and patient who, because of advanced age, has accumulated learned experience. Even more critically, it has been found that the member's older selves hold the "secrets" to the hitherto unarticulated social and medical health needs of this newly expanded population. These needs have a habit of gradually coming to the surface at a CCRC in the form of unexpected demands for service, causing unforeseen costs. Close member involvement with management can provide an early warning system, and allow effective planning for such costs.

How specifically is Villager input structured into PRC management? Two members of the elected Villager governing body sit in "as if" directors of the private corporations (PRC and the Medical Center) at the Company board meetings. The Villager Liaison Committee of three members, appointed by the Villager Board, meets weekly if not daily, with Core Team members, and monthly with Management Systems and as an integral part of the Team Assembly meetings. Committees of the Villagers, as stated earlier, meet monthly or as mutually agreed upon with each management service program. The Villager Board also has committees for numerous other functions such as activities planning, friendly visiting of lonely or ill members, library management, etc.—functions they so far wish to retain as their own, rather than management's concern. The Villager group "also appoints 19 cluster representatives," one for each of the 19 "neighborhoods" of apartments discussed earlier. These representatives assist both management and the Villagers in ensuring that cluster members are well, are visited when ill, are informed of ways to achieve their concerns within the Community, etc. Altogether, by recent estimate, more than 80% of the members are participating in one formalized Villager function or another during the course of the year.

The "Team Assembly" of Program Managers

In the daily life of the Village and the Medical Center, thirty baseline operating service programs have been defined. (See Exhibit 3.)

The managers of each of these programs meet monthly. The Core Team, the Villager Liaison Committee, and a representative of the Medical Center Patients Council are in attendance, as indicated above. This meeting is called Team Assembly. From the outset, the meeting has served to allow issues to surface for discussion in order to resolve conflict, clear up confusion over policy and procedure and increase staff interaction across programs. The Team Assembly has also heard lectures and training presentations and announcements of forthcoming PRC events. Lately, we see the Assembly intuitively follow the new "team mode" in the Community by breaking into ad hoc groups after the general meeting in order to strategize coming issues, e.g., a company-wide inventory, or a prospective decision on employee IRA strategies. In sum, this Assembly gives staff a chance to experience the interdisciplinary support PRC is working towards as a way to enhance quality of service.

The role of program managers and of Team Assembly will need to evolve further. Currently, the managers of five programs, all at the Medical Center, are asked to define their individual program plans with the same structural definitiveness that the five Core Team leaders demand of themselves in decision-making for their five over-arching areas of responsibility. Thus, like their Core Team bosses, these program managers must delineate for their programs:

1. A Statement of Philosophy, Policy and Policy-serving Procedure
2. A Client Multiphasic Assessment Plan
3. A Client Care Master Plan
4. A Financial Business Plan
5. A Marketing Plan
6. An Information Systems Plan for Research and Analysis

Ultimately, such in-depth planning will be expected of all thirty program managers (Exhibit 3).

What does such planning provide at PRC? A major challenge in such planning as an example, is to think through by way of these six program planning elements how to professionalize one's program along gerontological and geriatric lines. For some programs, this is relatively easy. Home health service or care of the ambulatory confused patient, for example, are PRC programs with obvious gerontological/geriatric input. Forming a Client Care Master Plan for them are part of the employee's professional training. Defining such a plan for service programs such as maintenance, however, requires of the employee a deeper than usual understanding of his task, clarity on how his task is different because he is at Pine Run, and an adjustment on his part to a care-giving point of view. How do effects of osteoporosis on body posture and movement shape the planning of scheduled apartment maintenance, for example? Employees must note the need to redesign with the passage of years the height of apartment cupboards for certain members. Maintenance has widened all PRC vehicle doors and added running boards and hand grips. Possibilities are endless. Awareness of these possibilities among program hands-on staff is the aim of a "Client Care Master Plan."

It should be noted that programs planned in this way can be managed both as semiautonomous professional units, and as business profit-and-loss building blocks forming an organization-wide financial and geriatric management plan. Both nonprofit and for-profit organizations when bent on improving operations, can use profits or surpluses creatively to expand program, but only where effective business plan management provides such surpluses.

Each program will ultimately have, as some now do, access to a work station terminal by which to tie-in with the main computer, a feature which expands data for accurate short and long-term forecasting. Both program director and the Villager Oversight Committee will have access through the program's terminal to the computer as technical expert which avoids secrecy in handling information and maximizes PRC's effort to be an "open book" management.

The Computer As Technical Executive

The computer, brought on line in Phase 2, becomes now in Phase 3 an efficient provider of technical information that releases PRC's staff for maximum human service effort. This is explained below.

The computer is the repository of primary data on PRC business activity, as well as of medical, social, biographic and financial data on all members and patients. A small accounting and programming staff in Management Systems who work as analysts, are now providing more effective reporting than the much larger bookkeeping staff of the past. As a matter of interest, the "overhead" cost of management, financial and information systems including the Core Team runs a little under 6% of gross revenue.

Financial watchdogging. Core Team receives final monthly and quarterly business plan financial statements fifteen days after the close of the previous month, accompanied by a cash forecast. In addition, an estimate of those final monthly outcomes, called a "Pretty Good Numbers Report" that has had 80% accuracy, is available to Core Team by the 20th of the month at hand, providing early warning on negative trends. The computer will increasingly make possible automatic forecasts of long-term results of existing trends, as well as sensitivity analyses and alternative option forecasts based on recommended changes on new sets of assumptions. Society tends to be suspicious of, if not hostile to, efforts at such quantitative control of "welfare work." We have found at PRC, however, that business plan reporting in accordance with generally accepted accounting principles (GAAP) actually enhances the "successful results" of social work. Not only does it document results, but it disciplines everyone in the organization against waste, and flags cost trends at once. Thus armed, the organization at once can seek cause and adjust and correct and thereby maximize the positive social program that can be provided with the available resources.

Toughminded forecasting. Furthermore, for an organization whose program is one of extensive long-term service guarantees, the long-term forecasts a computer allows become even more significant. PRC recognizes that one cannot be absolute in the prediction of future costs, but one can at least know, daily and as accurately as possible, that day's costs as a basis for that prediction. This in-depth monitoring by the computer at least allows maximum opportunity for planning and taking immediate action against negative trends whether these trends are 30 days or 20 years.

Forecasting morbidity and mortality. In addition to business activity, the PRC computer contains data describing members as individuals, as mentioned above. The plan is that there will ultimately be 1,000 bits of data on each person for whom PRC is responsible. Thus, it will be possible to forecast on a regular basis what PRC's unique collection of individuals as of a given time with their particular age, sex and social and health histories, will be likely to need in the arrangement of program services in the next 5 to 15 years. Again, the prediction cannot be absolute, but PRC will be more sensitively armed than without such predictions.

IV. Quality of Life at Pine Run Community[23]

What is life like in a community like Pine Run as compared to living in a broader community? When asked this question, PRC residents frequently commented on the psychosocial aspects of community life. Some of the comments are reproduced below.

"Family" and Friendship in a New Dimension

Mr. M. summarized the experience of life at Pine Run as "living in a very large family." People "pitch in." They care about each other. Other members added context. Friendships are closer at Pine Run than when working or in earlier retirement. Why? In part, there is more time for friendship because the community-in-miniature scale of life at Pine Run keeps friends close at hand, while the service supports preserve energy. In age, the loss of lifelong and cherished friends is constant, but at PRC one can retrieve closeness by finding an "ever-widening circle or a new friend." Most important, everyone is "in the same boat" of working at friendship. Having uprooted themselves and set up life in a new community, "we all make more effort here to reach out than we did in the 'stable' communities we came from." (Note that, in contrast to the image held by younger persons, a community of elders is sometimes seen by its members as ever-changing and open to new possibilities, while the broader community may be seen as "stable" if not somewhat stifling.)

"Unpleasant brothers and sisters", of course, there are. One does not like everyone. In a community like Pine Run, one knows one will have to deal with all members, however, on a day-to-day basis. Difficult individuals are difficult to avoid. Thus, members explained, "we try to be more open—enduring them, accepting them, sometimes finally enjoying them." That is the surprise. "We often find we have been depriving ourselves by being, initially, too judgmental." Interestingly, a defense strategy of avoidance can make sense in the broader community. At a center like Pine Run, however, where social boundaries are visible, a strategy of engagement in a difficult relationship provides a more successful defense.

Engagement is broadening. "Living at Pine Run is broadening," Mrs. B. explained. Like many, she had been a leader with wide interests throughout her life, but now faced physical ailments that were progressively narrowing her daily activities. Here, however, at dinner and elsewhere, she regains her sense of breadth and growth as she engages with ideas, opinions and recollections of other members. And she can maximize the leadership she still can offer because the arena for activity here is geographically tight.

Social Activity: Busier, With Meaning

Asked about life in their communities, CCRC dwellers comment: "We came expecting to retire, but we've never been busier."

Actually, as Mr. and Mrs. R. made clear, activities at Pine Run, as in most communities organized for the older old, are "more focused and selective" than in either the leisure retirement or the broader community. There one confronts "a newspaper full of activity" as compared to Pine Run's daily bulletin board.

But the scale apparently matches member energy and need. The busyness that members experience is "more fullfilling" because it realistically fills a true need. The activity is usually essential. Efforts for each other and for the Village are crucially important to the quality of life here, and every member knows it. "It's a community of which I am a full-fledged part," said one. "I'm not old here," said another. A third summed it up: "Our basic need to be truly needed is satisfied."

Some, like Mrs. T., were the gray eminences among younger friends in activities before coming here. Here they feel young again as their colleagues and friends are again their contemporaries. By contrast, others like Mrs. M., find that relationships here with the young people of the staff make them feel younger. "Here we see those younger people every day. We can build a closer relationship, provide counseling, be truly needed because of the frequency of contact not possible in the broader community."

For Miss S., leadership takes on new pleasure here. Everyone in a group is "on the same wavelength." One is a "leader among kindred spirits." One does "less explaining," less "bringing along" of group members who don't understand. "For the first time in my life, I am happy in leadership."

Facing Deterioration: A Range of Supports

Yes, it can be depressing at times to be among older people and see the deterioration. "On a street of mixed ages in the larger community, you're less aware of these problems than at Pine Run."

This is apparently outweighed, however, by the challenge and sense of new possibility that comes from seeing others overcome these difficulties. "One can't feel as sorry for oneself here," explained one relative newcomer. "I hesitated to walk from my apartment to the center, until I saw those with canes doing it." A new self-demand was born, her body grew stronger as she met that demand, and now "that walk is nothing." Others summed up, "One sees people getting out and doing things," as one could not in the larger community. Faced with these images, "one makes more effort here."

That effort is enabled and encouraged by the support from each other and from the staff. As we talked, a member joined us who had come up to the center from her apartment seeking distraction from the post-operative pain of a recent eye operation. A "buddy system" operates whereby members check each other daily. In the many "neighborhoods" on site, members are watchful to visit each other when sick, to draw out anyone who is isolated. Meantime, the home health and medical facility staff gives service and encouragement. "They make you keep trying. Without them I'd sit home and eat my milk toast."

The mutual and staff support is particularly enabling for the member who has to care for an invalid spouse. One no longer has to bear the full burden of care. One can "have daily input from 'doing your own thing' for a part of each day and thus get relief and a lift." And one gets support from other spouses near at hand who are "going through the same problems."

Ambivalences

Of course, there are trade offs. For everyone there is the adjustment to the inevitable influence of schedule. However a management tries, there still must be meal hours, scheduled bus runs, prescribed home health routines. New necessities for sharing arise, as with common washing machines that dot the campus and may not be free at the moment desired. All members experience a loss of control as the timelines and standards of others set the pace for such things as housekeeping and maintenance, even though they may have come to live here precisely because they could no longer personally handle the control of these arrangements.

For most, the first days here are hard. There are new relationships to build, new routines to grow used to. One of the most valuable Villager committees is the one devoted to easing these first weeks for new members.

But It All Feels "Normal"

"What is it like to live here? It feels normal," explained one couple. "We've been in residence long enough to feel 'set.' We have a feeling of belonging to the whole community."

In a telling phrase, that echoes the leading gerontologist Bernice Neugarten:[24] "You know, what feels normal changes as you move through life. In our thirties and forties it was our home on Long Island. In our sixties and early seventies it was Leisure Village. But now it is being here at Pine Run."

SUMMING UP[25]

PRC management structure has evolved over a nine-year period, and involved taking some perilous risks: the risk of setting up financial reporting standards in a predominantly non-profit field on a for-profit basis; the decision to institute at considerable expense comprehensive use of computer-based data gathering, control and reporting; and, finally the decision to allow management structures to evolve slowly through a reciprocal learning experience of open engagement with members and patients as if they too were the founders, managers, and care-givers at PRC, not merely the consumers.

Risk-taking often leads to growth. Members, patients and management have done a great deal of growing at PRC. PRC Villagers have grown into a hardy stock of renewed survivors, aided by having a voice in their future and in the CCRC gerontological designs that provide them with a special kind of efficiency of living that continues to make longitudinal sense even as they become very, very old. Management, meanwhile, has grown through the development of a team focus, business management discipline, computer technology, and open dialogue with those it is serving in a dynamic gerontological milieu.

Pine Run, and other communities like it, are products of the ideals of self reliance at advanced age that abound in our country today. A common misunderstanding of these communities is to castigate them as "age segregation." A more sensitive understanding recognizes that the American tradition, starting with the first landing at Plymouth, has often been to meet crises by self-sorting into corporate bodies of like-minded people, supporting one another in a single community, perhaps as a religious commune or in private volunteer striving.

It is not surprising that this same tradition, confronting the 20th century crisis of large numbers of long living elders, should find it normal and enriching to meet that crisis with the concept of the continuing care retirement community—a community that brings together not only those of like mind, but of like age.

What has emerged for PRC management is a new freedom to grow continuously and professionally in the field of aging, with its clients who are over 70, who have "been there," who have earned their way, and who are willing to share ideas on how to use tomorrow as a practical future.

REFERENCES

1. Winklevoss, Howard E. and Powell, Alwyn V., *Continuing Care Retirement Communities: An Empirical, Financial and Legal Analysis,* Homewood, Illinois: Richard D. Irwin, Inc., 1984, pp. 288, 290.

2. Ibid., pp. 9, 289-290, and chapters 4-9.

3. Moyer, Paul R., M.D., *Cash Flow In a Life Care Community, A Stochastic Model,* Doylestown, Pennsylvania: LCSA, Incorporated Library, July 31, 1979.

4. Dorris, James R., *Consumers Guide to Independent Living for Older Americans: The Life Care Alternative,* Doylestown, Pa.: LCSA, Incorporated, 1979. Also, Winklevoss, p. 28.

5. Bourliere, F., *Gerontology Before and After 1950: The Final Accounting,* Lecture before the Belgium Society of Gerontology, Summer 1977. (Doylestown, Pa.: Elliott translation, LCSA, Incorporated Library).

6. Hayflick, Leonard, *Abstract: Biological Aspects of Human Aging,* Symposium on Multi-dimensional Diagnostics and Therapy in Gerontopsychiatry, Cologne, Germany, July 19-21, 1981.

7. Reis, Werner, *Studien zum Biologishen Alter,* Berlin, D.D.R.: Akademie Verlag, 1982.

8. Hazan, Haim, *The Limbo People: A Study of the Constitution of the Time Universe Among the Aged,* London: Routledge and Kegan Paul, 1980.

9. Rautenberg, E.L., *Ethnocultural Factors in Delivery of Health Services,* Paper presented at the 110th Annual Meeting of the American Public Health Association, Montreal, Canada, November, 1981.

10. Rosenmayr, L., "Progress and Unresolved Problems in Sociogerontological Theory," *Aktuelle Gerontologie,* Stuttgart: George Thieme Verlag, 1979, Vol. 9, pp. 197-205.

11. Rosenmayr, L., *What is the Social Aspect of Aging,* Symposium (supra at #6).

12. Thomae, H. (Ed), *Patterns of Aging: Findings from the Bonn Longitudinal Study of Aging,* Basle-New York: Kargel, 1976.

13. Birren, James and Schroots, J.J.F., *The Psychological Point of View Toward Human Aging and Adaptability,* Paper presented at the 9th International Congress of Social Gerontology (ICSG), Quebec, Canada, August, 1980.

14. Erikson, E.H., *Identity and the Life Cycle,* New York: W.W. Norton & Co., 1979.

15. Lienert, G.A., Gebert, A., Kohnen, R., *Multivariate Psychology,* Symposium (supra at #6).

16. Pelicier, Yves, *Modeles Psychopathologiques et Capacite D'Arbitrage Des Contraintes Chez le Sujet Age,* Paper presented at the 9th ICSG (supra at #13).

17. Pfeiffer, Eric, "Survival in Old Age: Physical, Psychological and Social Correlates of Longevity", *Journal of the American Geriatric Society,* Vol. 18(4), pp. 273-285, April, 1970.

18. Galbreath, Jay, *Designing Complex Organizations,* Reading, Massachusetts: Addison-Wesley Publishing Co., 1973.

19. Kouzes, J.M. and Mico, P.R., "Domain Theory: An Introduction to Organizational Behavior in Human Service Organizations", *Journal of Applied Behavioral Science,* 1979, pp. 449-469.

20. Mouzalis, Nicos P., *Organization and Bureaucracy: An Analysis of Modern Theories,* New York: Aldine Publishing Company, 1967.

21. Sashkin, Marshall, "Changing Toward Participative Management Approaches: A Model and Methods", *Academy of Management Review,* Vol. 1(3), pp. 75-86, July, 1976.

22. Davies, Stanley M. and Lawrence, Paul R., *Matrix,* Reading, Massachusetts: Addison-Wesley Publishing Company, 1977.

23. See also Schwartz, Doris, F.A.A.N., Resident of Foulkeways, Gwynedd, Pa., Testimony at U.S. Senate Special Committee on Aging Hearing on Continuing Care Retirement Communities, May 25, 1983.

24. Neugarten, Bernice L. and Hagestad, Gunhild O., "Age and the Life Course" in Binstock, Robert H. and Shanas, Ethel (Eds.), *Handbook of Aging and the Social Sciences,* New York: Van Nostrand Reinhold Co., 1976.

25. Selznick, P., *Leadership in Administration: A Sociological Interpretation,* New York: Harper and Row, 1957.

PART IV:
BACKGROUND INFORMATION ON THE SITUATION IN NEW YORK STATE

Introduction to Part IV

The papers in this section attempt to describe the current political climate which is unfavorable to continuing care retirement communities to be established in New York State.

In *Chapter 7*, George Warner traces the background history of current regulations in regard to the construction of new health care facilities. He explains that the original thrust of legislation in this field was aimed toward securing the quality of health services provided as well as the long range financial stability of the service providers. Within this context evolved the prohibition against pre-paid life contracts in the health care aspect of the long term care spectrum which now effectively prohibits retirement communities in New York State to include prepaid health services in their residents' agreements.

In *Chapter 8*, Corinne Plummer deals with New York State policies in regard to life care contracts from the vantage point of social services. She explains the problems involved when oversight is assumed by many different agencies on various levels of long term care. She also describes the role and responsibility of the Department of Social Services in regard to adult homes and the problems involved in certification of facilities which offer residential as well as health care services.

In *Chapter 9*, Lloyd Nurick offers a rationale for the political

99

climate that seems to be opposed to the establishment of CCRCs in New York State. However, he observes that changing public opinion and economic realities seem to be effective in turning policy makers toward more favorable consideration and acceptance of this long term care alternative for the retirees of the state of New York. He also discusses the issues of regulation, sources of funding and sponsorship of future CCRCs.

Chapter 7

Policies on Retirement Communities in New York State: Historical Background and Current Status From the Vantage Point of Health Care

George M. Warner

The purpose of this chapter is to describe what the background was, and the events were that led to the prohibition against life-care contracts and similar arrangements in the health care part of the continuing care spectrum in New York State.

On May 25, 1964 Governor Rockefeller appointed a Committee on Hospital Costs chaired by the distinguished Marion Folsom from Rochester, New York. Mr. Folsom previously had served as HEW's Secretary under President Eisenhower in addition to functioning as an executive of a major multi-national business corporation and establishing a fine reputation for his "volunteer" health and social welfare activities in New York State. The charges to that Committee basically were: to examine the rapidly rising costs of hospital and other health care services (this has a familiar ring to it) to try to determine what some of the causative factors were; and, to recommend to the Governor and both Houses of the New York State Legislature moves that might be made and actions that might be taken to slow these rapidly spiraling costs. The Folsom Committee, which it came to be called, turned in its initial report on April 9, 1965. Its final report was delivered on December 15, 1965. In its preliminary as well as final reports the Committee indicated that it

George M. Warner, M.D., Special Health Care Advisor, Health Facilities Standards and Surveillance, State of New York Department of Health, Albany, N.Y.

101

had examined many of the reasons underlying rapidly increasing health care costs and advised that legislative, gubernatorial and public attention be turned to and focused on nine major problem areas.

In April 1965, in a very unusual bipartisan move, the upper and lower houses of the State Legislature, with full support of the Governor's Office and several State agencies, enacted legislation to carry out the major recommendations of the Folsom Committee. That legislation was signed in early summer of 1965, shortly before President Johnson signed the Medicare and Medicaid legislation, which were to become effective the following year, on July 1, 1966. We thus had the birth in New York State of Article 28 of the Public Health Law and a number of complementary changes in State insurance law, State social welfare law and other laws.

One of the basic three thrusts of the new Article 28 (provisions of which were to become effective on February 1 of the following year, 1966), was to create a central focal point for standards for the quality of care in New York State. The New York State Health Department was named as that focal point.

Second, Article 28 created authority at the State level to establish rates for payment for hospital and other services and located the focal point for establishing those rates in one agency at the State level, the Department of Health. Rates, by the way, that were to be set were to apply to all instances in which public monies were to be used to pay for care. Included in the definition of "public monies" were then, and still are, Blue Cross monies or monies expended for care by quasi-public insurance corporations as well as state and local tax monies.

The third major thrust of the legislation was to create Statewide and regional controls over health care resources so that they would be evenly and fairly distributed throughout the State and so that the resources would not be greater than the estimated need for health care services.

Article 28 utilized the word "hospital" in a much broader context than that term is ordinarily used. "Hospitals" and "hospital services" were defined to include a variety of different kinds and levels of providers, including support services that were furnished through those providers to the public. Nursing homes, independent clinics, home care agencies, etc. were swept in under the "hospital" rubric.

In 1965 the Folsom Committee pointed out that, with the then awesome spiraling of hospital costs, within several years it was quite possible that acute community general hospital care might even reach the astounding cost of $100 per day (!) and that the public might have to be concerned with hospital stays that would cost at least $1,000! It is now nineteen years later. We all know what the interim story has been and now is with regard to hospital costs.

The long-term care portion of the health care spectrum was not singled out and given any great prominence either in the Folsom report or in the formulation of the Article 28 legislation. The major focus was on the general hospital part of the health care scene, which at that time was consuming by far the majority of the health care dollar. It is only in the years since then that we have come to realize the significance of the long-term care part of the scene.

On signature of Article 28 into law, the New York State Health Department promptly reorganized (as all bureaucracies have a habit of doing from time-to-time) to take on its rather awesome responsibilities. The then Bureau of Chronic Diseases and Geriatrics reorganized into two units; a new Bureau of Long Term Care, which I had the fortunate pleasure (or load, or task) of heading; and an Adult Health and Geriatrics Bureau, which continued to work in multiphasic screening and in the preventive medicine arena in geriatrics.

The job of the Long Term Care Bureau, in the early Fall of 1965, was to begin to draft standards which might be applicable to that category of institutions which we at the State bureaucracy level knew at the time as "nursing homes." A number of preparatory activities were involved. We obtained and reviewed nursing home standards from forty-two other States. We had been working with the then Board of Social Welfare in drafting what were going to be proposed as new Statewide standards to be administered pre Article 28, by the Board of Social Welfare and the Department of Social Services. We also had been guiding the standards activities of sixteen city and county health jurisdictions that had their own nursing home codes that were administered at the local level under the State-aid to local health programs. New York City, by the way, had its own standards and enforcement program for controlling quality of care and safety of the environment in all the proprietary hospitals and nursing homes.

So we had the benefits of reviewing standards and experiences with them from other States, from New York City, from cities and counties in other parts of New York State and at a Statewide level. We then began the prolonged and difficult job of drafting a new set of requirements applicable to the nursing home type providers.

Fairly early in the drafting process, we developed review procedures that included presentations and discussions about each successive draft, as it was completed, with representatives of the major parties which might have key concerns about and interests in the standards. These included, of course, the provider organizations, of which there were two major Statewide associations at the time, and the major provider professions (organizations of the medical profession, the nursing profession, the social workers, rehabilitation therapists and others). I would remind us that at that point in time when Article 28 became effective (only five months before Medicare and Medicaid) in New York State, there were some 42,500 nursing home beds (a count which was not terribly accurate, by the way), all of them at what we would now call the SNF or skilled nursing facility level of care. There was no recognition of the level of care we now call ICF or HRF.

Our early findings in looking at these 42,500 beds in about 700 facilities were that over one-half of the beds were in facilities that were not suitable for long-range use. That is, the patients were housed in buildings which were structurally deficient, not in conformance with existing fire safety standards or with other kinds of environmental requirements. The resource of suitable nursing home facilities was a very slim one, indeed—especially in light of the estimated needs at that time. Estimated needs for long-term care beds and services, by the way, were at an even higher level then than they are now, some years later (I believe I recall that estimates at that time were for 120,000 or more beds, whereas the planners now estimate a need for about 105,000 beds). So, one-half of the existing resource was not suitable for use for much longer than several years after the Article 28 program began and to meet the needs that might be accelerated not long after that by the benefits anticipated from Title XVIII and Title XIX of the Federal Law.

In the process of drafting the quality of care standards, it became clear that other provisions of Article 28 also had to be examined very carefully. Standards would have to conform to cost concerns and perhaps to other requirements that were not necessarily related directly to the quality and safety of buildings and environments or to the quality of care of patients, goals of Article 28.

One of the provisions which required continuing attention was that sponsors intending to construct new facilities, to add beds to or renovate existing facilities or to change ownership must meet several tests in order to secure approval at the State level to take those actions (of building new plants, changing ownership, etc.).

Such sponsors had to meet a "public need" or a Certificate of Need test (a resource control requirement). They had to meet a "Character, Competence and Standing in the community" test (i.e., assurances had to be provided that the individuals intending to participate as sponsors and the overall sponsor organizations would have predictable competence to construct, operate and otherwise provide health care services efficiently and in conformance with State requirements). And third, and very focal to the interest of this volume and the Conference on which it is based, there had to be evidence of financial feasibility of the project that was being planned, whether it be a new facility or changes in an existing one.

The actual language, which remains in Article 28 today, basically said that the anticipated future sources of revenue had to be sufficient to meet future operating costs. The rationale for including such language legislatively is a little difficult to trace. One suspects that it was part of the overall philosophy that emanated basically from the Folsom Report that was the foundation of Article 28—namely, that legislative and executive leadership people in this State wanted a health care resource for the future which would be reliable, which could be counted on to provide at least reasonable quality of care and which could provide effectively, at reasonable costs and reliably over the anticipated service or life span of each of the facilities in the resource.

In arriving at the new standards, therefore, we (the drafters) and those who were engaged in the review processes had to be continuously cognizant of this requirement that anticipated future sources of revenue must be estimated to be adequate to meet future operating costs of the facilities. As a result of this requirement we drafted into the earliest versions of the Code a very simple provision which remains unchanged to date.

This provision, germane to the interest of this Conference, is the one that did say and does say "*the operator shall not enter into any contract or agreement with a patient, resident, next of kin and/or sponsor for life care of the patient or resident.*" That phraseology, with almost no change, is present today.

In our meetings with the provider organizations we identified a clear reason for creating that phraseology, it having become quite clear in the Winter of 1965 and early Spring of 1966 that facilities engaged in life-care contract arrangements were already beginning to have some serious financial difficulties because of the rapidly increasing costs of health facility care. Many of those life-care contracts included guarantees of coverage, not only for residential care on the premises of the then loosely described long-term care facilities, but also for care in the infirmary or sick bay sections of such facilities and, where medically necessary, even in some instances for hospital care. Many of the arrangements or contracts that patients or residents had made with sponsors of long-term care complexes were quite comprehensive and did, in some instances, include assurances/guarantees that contractees would be guaranteed hospital care and that payments for that hospital care would be made by the sponsors. To our fiscal and other co-drafting personnel, these kinds of arrangements were of such nature as to cause great concern for the future financial stability of the facilities.

A second stimulus came from the organizations of the providers themselves. In 1965 and 1966 there were two major Statewide organizations: the New York Association of Homes for the Aging and the New York State Nursing Home Association. The New York Association of Homes for the Aging, a fairly young organization at that time, included in its membership many of the leading voluntary non-profit institutions. The New York State Nursing Home Association represented most of the proprietary facilities. Representatives of the New York Association of Homes for the Aging, in our many and frequent meetings with them, brought directly to our attention the fact that some of their members were already beginning to suffer from the financial burden of life-care contracts which their endowments and incomes from endowments and gifts from other sources could no longer sustain. Therefore, they requested that we draft and adopt in Code the language that would help their members deal with such problems in the future.

So the original language (which prohibited life-care contracts) and subsequent language (which prohibited advance payments for more than three months at a time) was a product of two forces. One was the requirement of Article 28 that facilities must have and provide some assurances of long range financial viability as a part of the State's health care resources. Second, that whatever arrangements were made for payments to providers for services, these arrangements must be financially sound and ethically acceptable. They should not be barriers hindering access to and use by those needing health services or threats to the financial viability of institutions.

Since the State Hospital Code requirements went into effect on February 1, 1966, there have been no reasons to change the prohibition against life-care contracts in the health care aspects of the long term care spectrum. For emphasis, we should underline "*in the health care aspects of the long term care spectrum.*" No long term health care facility, regardless of its sponsorship, presumably has been permitted to enter into such contracts since that time. With the still increasing costs of the Residential Health Care Facility portion of the health care spectrum and with anticipations that SNF and HRF care costs are going to increase further (because the patient populations are sicker, are being admitted earlier from hospitals, have more complex chronic illness conditions, and are increasingly older and more frail patients), there are no reasons to anticipate that the costs of long-term health care are going to level off or decrease in our foreseeable future. Therefore, to retain these prohibitions against the financial arrangements that in fact may and could become disastrous to sponsoring institutions does seem to make good sense.

One footnote is that, in several instances, facilities that were beginning to encounter serious financial difficulties in the mid 1960s in trying to adhere to the terms of their existing life-care contracts with their residents sought relief through the regulatory avenue. They came to us and said, "Can you help? We are paying out funds which are far beyond our capacity to pay in order to adhere to the provisions of these contracts. Can you, New York State, prohibit us from continuing to honor these contracts and thus be forced into bankruptcy?" We, with good advice from our attorneys, were forced to say, "No, we cannot." "We can, through State Hospital Code requirements and with statutory backing prohibit new arrangements of this sort. But we can do nothing about the contracts that are already in effect. That will have to be a matter that you will have to settle with your residents and through whatever administrative and legal avenues you have." I do recall, by the way, that Bethel Methodist Home (located in Ossining, not far north of New York City) was one of the earliest to test this matter in court. I think, if I recall, they lost their attempt to modify the life-care contracts that that facility had with some of its residents for the nursing home portion of care.

So that is the background. I think it important that we keep in mind that there were these major forces, behind the scenes and in the open, that led to very serious financial and other considerations about the efficacy of life-care arrangements in health care. The huge emerging problems at that time were spiraling hospital costs, mostly in the general hospital arena. Recommendations were that the State on behalf of its residents must exert controls over the supply and distribution of its health care resources. There were deepseated concerns about protecting consumers of health services by creating and implementing minimum standards for quality of care and for quality and safety of health facility environments statewide. There were concerns that the costs of care should be properly and fully paid for, but also and at later points, that costs and payments should meet the test of efficient delivery of services. These and others were and continue to be the very important forces that led to the kinds of prohibitions and understandings about life-care contracts that now exist here in New York State.

Chapter 8

Policies on Retirement Communities in New York State: Historical Background and Current Status From the Vantage Point of Social Services

Corinne Plummer

It is important to keep in mind that New York State has yet to address continuing care, particularly the concept of continuing care communities, as a distinct entity, although it does have policies governing narrow areas, such as admission to residential health care facilities (RHCFS), and Medicaid eligibility. Some of the issues relative to continuing care, and particularly to life-care contracts, have been raised in a number of State programs, but the State response has been, admittedly, piecemeal. The Private Housing Finance Law and the Not-for-Profit Corporation Law impose certain conditions on organizations which propose to offer housing accommodations for the aged or disabled. Both Social Services and Health Law set standards for the provision of certain services that are integral to the delivery of continuing care. Each agency also certifies and oversees facilities which respond to particular segments of the care continuum. Despite extensive involvement in most of the individual elements of continuing care communities, public consideration of promotion of continuing care retirement communities, of coordinated oversight, or of the role of public funding in such settings has been limited.

The New York State Department of Social Service (DSS) is re-

Corinne Plummer, Deputy Commissioner, Division of Adult Services, New York State Department of Social Services.

109

sponsible for the certification and supervision of adult homes. These are residential facilities, nearly 500 in number with 20,000 beds, which provide personal care and supervision to dependent adults who do not need the nursing supervision available in health-related and skilled nursing facilities. The Department of Social Services is also responsible for setting standards and determining eligibility, through local departments of social services, for Medicaid. Continuing care, particularly, life-care contracts, has been an issue in each of these areas.

The history of life-care and the contracts for such care in residential facilities is briefly described below. Not-for-profit organizations in New York State, frequently church-related but sometimes established by a family or individual, have been responding to the life-care needs of aged and indigent persons for well over a hundred and fifty years. Some of these have become very sophisticated multilevel facilities, others have remained as 20-bed-rest homes, and most others fall somewhere in between. Historically, the first responsibility of overseeing such facilities fell to the Board of Social Welfare. Dr. Warner (see previous chapter) wrote about the impact of Article 28 and the clear distinction required between nursing facilities and adult homes. For DSS purposes, this and the introduction of Medicare and Medicaid in the late 60s, with strict standards for federal participation in the public funding of nursing homes, are critical benchmarks.

Facilities, including a number of organizations which then offered life-care contracts, had to be reclassified as either Medicaid-fundable or not. The decisions were obviously made on levels of care to be offered, but the match between the physical plant and the fairly rigorous environmental standards for federal funding was also considered. As Dr. Warner mentioned, a significant number of facilities were designated non-conforming and were slated to close or be phased out. A number of not-for-profit facilities were designated homes for the aged under the supervision of the Department of Social Services and the Board of Social Welfare, rather than nursing facilities under the Health Department. Initial planning and regulation permitted these adult homes to maintain infirmaries which were to be jointly supervised by Health and the Board but, like many cooperative oversight agreements, that joint effort was not realized.

Unlike the Department of Health, the Board of Social Welfare stood essentially silent on the issue of life-care contracts. Although no Board policy was articulated on life care, it did take note of the hearing decisions on Medicaid, which will be described below. Although some Homes for the Aged decided on their own to cease offering such contracts, others did not. In 1977, when the responsibility for certification and supervision of adult care facilities was transferred from the Board of Social Welfare to the Department of Social Services, between 30 and 40 facilities which had life-care residents were identified and at least 10 of those were still admitting new residents under life-care agreements.

This posed interesting problems for the DSS. First there was, and is today, the level of care issue. Adult homes certified by the Department of Social Services are by statutory definition non-medical facilities. They are not permitted by statute to admit or retain persons who ought to be cared for in a health-related or skilled nursing facility. Rather than change past practice or take on the expense of care in a medical facility, many adult homes simply went into, or continued, the provision of nursing care on a small scale. Infirmaries and small nursing units are still common in some not-for-profit adult homes, especially those with a life-care population. The problems of regulatory oversight have been complicated by the potential impact that abrupt closure of such nursing units would have on the individual residents and the financial viability of the home.

Since 1977, the DSS has actively discouraged facilities from writing life-care agreements. With the understanding, if not the backing of the NY State Assn. of Homes for the Aged, DSS has taken concrete action to prohibit the execution of any new admission agreements which provide that a resident may receive care for life *in the adult home* should the resident require continuous medical or nursing services. We have also limited the continued residence of individuals with current life-care contracts whose needs cannot be met within the facility. We took this step for several reasons: the limits imposed by law on our regulatory authority; social services staff simply does not have the expertise to monitor the provisions of health services; because of our concern for resident care and basic life safety.

In retelling history, it is necessary to shift to the other program within the Department which is germane to continuing care communities—Medicaid. As Dr. Warner noted (previous chapter) one of the reasons the Health Department prohibited life-care contracts was in reaction to the now familiar and very real problem of organizational default or insolvency. In the past, at least in New York's experience, some organizations which promised life-care at set fees or even with escalator-clauses were unable to meet their contractual obligations to the resident. Many have attempted to solve these problems by seeking Medicaid funding for individual residents. This has been especially true in instances where adult home residents under life-care contracts need nursing home care and the adult home has chosen to transfer them.

Under the Medicaid regulations, a life-care contract is to be considered a resource for purposes of determining eligibility. The resources of the *home* are considered available to meet the needs of the individual unless it can be demonstrated that the home is unable to fulfill its obligation. This position has been tested in the courts and generally upheld with the exception of one case (Episcopal v. Toia) which held that a contract which explicitly provides for care only while the resident remains in the facility may be considered to end if transfer to an appropriate setting is made.

There is, however, a procedure under which a facility may require the Department to suspend consideration of the life-care contract as a resource. In order to do this, the facility must submit financial records detailing the degree of loss for the home overall. The Department, in turn, consults with the Department of Health, and may then grant Medicaid eligibility. In such situations, which must be reassessed annually, a resident is entitled to Medicaid reimbursement for medical service only up to the resident's pro-rate share of the facility's losses. For example, if 10 residents have suspended contracts and the facility has operating losses of $10,000, the first $1,000 of *each* resident's allowable medical expenses are MA reimbursable. Apart from the merits of such a policy it has obviously functioned as a major disincentive to the growth of traditionally financed life-care communities.

This is a brief factual description of the Department's past and current involvement with life-care contracts. We support efforts to carefully examine the place of these communities and the type and degree of government involvement warranted. Consumer protection, level of care, joint oversight, State regulation and other important issues are explored in depth in other sections of this volume. The results should help New York look closely at the potential role of Continuing Care Retirement Communities. The Department of Social Services stands by the decisions made to date, but it is open to a public policy discussion of where to go from here. The failure to reexamine old policy in light of new opportunities could have serious consequences for the ability of the public and private sectors, in partnership, to respond to the needs and preferences of our elderly and disabled. Thus these proceedings are intended to make a significant contribution to that work.

Chapter 9

The Prospect for the Future of Continuing Care Retirement Communities in New York State

Lloyd Nurick

Three themes seem to run through many of the papers in this volume which have implications for New York State policy. The first one is the element of provision of services. Second, there seem to be very positive feelings now toward continuing care retirement communities, which was not the case earlier, and third, there is a great concern over protection of the resident or the potential resident of such communities. New York is the only state in the union with prohibitions against life care through all health care levels—one state out of 50.

This may be the case because of the unique structuring of society in New York. New York is the only state that is similar to the Western European welfare state. Welfare state is not meant as a pejorative phrase. New York seems to look eastward to Europe for the system for structuring its programming for residents. It is possible also to look northward to Canada and find a similar situation. But you find almost nothing in the way of similar social programming throughout the rest of the country.

This tendency may come from the history of New York which was a "melting pot." The immigrants from Europe landed in New York and came together in social groupings which, to a large degree, were social groupings out of Eastern Europe, perhaps out of the socialist developments of the late 19th and early 20th centuries. These immigrants believed in group programs and they believed in government support systems and regulation. Those people who

Lloyd Nurick, Director, New York Association of Homes and Services for the Aging, Albany, New York.

115

were more entrepreneurial, more independent in their way of life, moved west via the wagon trains and other means of moving. Those who remained were social in nature to the extent that they looked toward and created governments that would provide social services for them.

There are a few other states that have similar patterns, namely Massachusetts, Minnesota, and Wisconsin, probably for similar reasons. But New York probably epitomizes the welfare state in the United States.

This means that the attitudes towards service in New York State focus on government regulation and government-initiated programming. This also means that there is a focus on equal access to services. Thus, the concept of selective living arrangements for the middle classes may be antithetical to the social and political perceptions of most New Yorkers. This may well be what continuing care communities represent to most New Yorkers and the legislative and governmental bodies that represent them.

George Warner (Chapter 7) and Corinne Plummer (Chapter 8) described the history of what happened in New York State to precipitate the elimination of life care contracts. The welfare state approach outlined above may have had as much to do with eliminating life care contracts as the specific pragmatic situations and moments in time when these policies were promulgated.

However, New York seems to be changing because of new economic circumstances, caused by both federal and state conditions. With New York's new emphasis on a strong economic base, continuing care communities may offer some benefits.

Thus, New Yorkers seem to be warming to the notion of life care communities perhaps because they represent a source of revenue to the state. Depending on how life care communities cater to their client group, there may be taxes available. In addition, the new employees in the communities in which they will be located will be paying additional taxes. And these continuing care communities will provide jobs for local communities that may need them.

The timeliness of the continuing care retirement community may also be a factor in changing the predisposition of New Yorkers towards them. There have been dramatic changes in the long term care system in New York and around the country which have been addressed in this volume. These changes seem to revolve around (1) decrease in need for intermediate care facilities (2) enlightened legislation and (3) the possibility of by-passing the certificate of need (CON) process.

There is a great expansion on the ends of the continuum of care—housing and skilled nursing—with reduction in usage of the domiciliary and health related facility. There are five or six reasons for this happening at this time:

First, the growth of housing for the elderly like 202 projects and other housing types with congregate services is preventing people from entering middle level institutions. There is much talk about a continuum of care. But to some extent it seems that when you capture a person at a given level, that person tends to remain at that level until something traumatic occurs at which point the person enters a skilled nursing facility, probably after a period of hospitalization. That person does not really move through a continuum; he or she jumps from wherever he or she was along the continuum to the most intense level of care.

Second, better health and medical care generally has lessened the need for the intermediate care facilities such as the HRF and domiciliary care facility.

Third, and very important, the dramatic growth in outreach services, particularly in New York State, has lessened the need for intermediate level facilities. A figure released about a year ago by the N.Y. State Health Planning Commission indicates that from about 1975 to 1979, the increase in home care services was approximately 69%. Thus, with the advent of long term home health care programs, day care programs and such recent innovations as respite care, frail elderly people are able to remain home for longer periods of time.

Fourth, the modern American has become more independent and may be unwilling to conform, a requirement of living in a group setting. Health related and domiciliary facility settings are group settings, meaning that: one goes to meals at the same time as others; one does not cook one's own meals; and one has to live according to the lifestyle in that facility no matter how much the facility professes to encourage independence. The average person with a three bedroom home or six room apartment in New York City who can simply cook a TV dinner whenever he or she wants to, or do whatever he wants when he wants to, is not going to look toward a group living arrangement as one of choice. Usually, the decision to be institutionalized involves very little choice.

Fifth, people are living longer and they are living longer together with spouses. As a result, they may be able to support each other and may thereby reduce the need for institutional facilities and increase the need for community-type retirement settings.

Sixth, it is possible that the nursing home scandals of the mid-70s, and the continuing negative attitudes towards institutions conveyed by the media may have caused people to be "disattracted," if there is such a word, to long term care institutions until there is absolutely no other alternative.

To repeat, the middle level of care seems to be deteriorating to some degree. Thus, the continuing care retirement community seems to be filling a gap at that middle level. It seems to provide housing, nursing care when needed, as well as outreach programs to people in their own new homes. This certainly is a more appealing approach than middle level institutional care as represented by HRFs, ICFs and DCFs.

As for the theme of offering protection to the resident, there is the feeling that this can occur through legislation which protects the consumer, the provider and the state. As mentioned above, in New York, nothing happens without a law. So, continuing care retirement communities will inevitably come under state regulation.

A number of questions arise concerning this last point:

One, who should regulate? One or several agencies? A single agency is always best for a control mechanism. But if it is one agency then which one should it be? The Insurance Department? The Housing and Community Renewal Division? The Attorney General who is very active in contract law and in consumer law? The Division of Consumer Affairs? The Department of Social Services? The Department of Health? These questions need to be answered before policies regarding continuing care communities can be formulated.

Two, is there a need for a certificate of need process? This question raises a number of other issues. Let us assume that the argument is in favor of a certificate of need process especially if Medicaid dollars are to be used for the purchase of long term care services. Medicaid dollars are state, federal and local dollars. Public money is being spent, which at the moment is not open ended, thus leading to a certificate of need process which inhibits the growth of beds. If one assumes that there must be equal access to services for the "haves" and the "have nots," which was mentioned above as a philosophy of New York State, then a certificate of need process is necessary. Basically this limits services for both the rich and the poor.

However, it is possible to alter our view. Thus, those who "have" shall have unlimited access to nursing home beds and other institutional resources which they purchase while those who "have not'' and whose services are purchased by the government may be thought of as not being entitled to these types of services. Special services may be developed for them.

Of course, the certificate of need process must take into consideration the impact of a life care community on other services in a community such as the local fire department, police department, hospital and physician supply, etc.

Perhaps it is possible to do away with the CON process. If there is no involvement of public funds, no Medicaid, no SSI, no 202, no HUD resources, perhaps there is no need for CON. Perhaps if people can band together and do things on their own with their own finances, and guarantee the government that there will be no government involvement in the future, there should be no need to go through the CON process. We have to consider the fact that a continuing care retirement community is not necessarily a local group which is measured by a bed needs methodology according to county size. People may be coming to these communities from all over: in fact, the bed needs methodology for long term care presently exempts special groups such as the Masons and the Odd Fellows, which have statewide or broader constituencies.

This point of view clearly runs counter to current New York State ideology. We seem to be describing a free market situation, so we may be arguing against not only certificate of need, but against regulation as a whole. This may be unacceptable in New York State.

On the other hand, it may be possible to use federal and state dollars for life care communities. It may be possible for Medicaid to buy into them. Thus, if you open a life care community and Medicaid wishes to put down $50,000 and pay a monthly fee or finance a social health maintenance organization (S/HMO), is there not room for this within the continuing care retirement community?

As an alternative to the S/HMO, how about an end payment when the person requires admission into the medical part of the community? Medicaid could buy in at that point if personal resources are spent or about to be used up so that it becomes a supplement for private payment. If it is possible to consider family supplements for Medicaid payments, why not reverse it? Why not consider Medicaid supplements for family payments? Thus, a resident can be maintained in a continuing care community in the best manner possible without having to pay 100% of the cost.

Presumably in New York State, there will be government intervention at some level in any sort of program development that could potentially benefit or harm the state as a whole. If there is government intervention, at the least there must be coordination among government agencies, in order to allow facilities that are going to be continuing care retirement communities to become functioning organizations without having to go through a series of processes which takes years and delays services which can benefit the frail elderly who cannot wait.

If such communities are allowed in New York State, who should sponsor them? There is much discussion about this issue in this volume, reflecting a concern of conference participants. Here, I would like to recommend for New York State only voluntary sponsorship and operation of continuing care retirement communities. This recommendation is made for the following reasons: (1) there seems to be evidence that there is a need for a community or religious base to improve the chance of marketing success in the field; (2) pressure by the sponsoring entities helps to assure quality and excellence of care; (3) in Pennsylvania, it has been found that facilities without problems tend to be denominational, facilities with major problems tend to be developer originated; (4) although problems can occur in voluntary communities, such as Pacific Homes, voluntary groups have and can support these financial difficulties. In the case of Pacific Homes, the Methodist churches of America got together and contributed $21 million to support the continuation of Pacific Homes. In other than a voluntary situation, there might not be that capability.

To conclude, based on my own observations and the conference proceedings, it would seem that for New York State (1) continuing care retirement communities are feasible; (2) continuing care retirement communities probably should be tried and (3) continuing care retirement communities probably will develop, one way or another there, with or without legislation.

PART V:
LOOKING TOWARD THE FUTURE: ISSUES TO BE CONSIDERED AND RECOMMENDATIONS FOR ACTION

Introduction to Part V

The papers in this section are edited versions of workshop reports as they were originally written and presented by the workshop recorders to the plenary session at the conclusion of the conference. Workshop chairmen and panelists are listed as co-authors.

The workshops met twice on 2 different days dealing with the same topic each time, thus giving conference participants the opportunity to take part in the discussion of two different topics. For the purpose of this volume, an attempt has been made to condense the panel presentations, discussions and recommendations into one report.

The conference program included five workshops on the following themes: Public Policy Issues, Legal Issues and Barriers, Financial and Actuarial Aspects, Programmatic and Operational Problems and Consumer Interests. The following chapters represent some of the ideas and recommendations brought forward during the workshop sessions. Please note that there is no separate report on the workshop on Consumer Interests. However the recommendations formulated by that workshop's participants are included in the report on Public Policy.

All of the reports reflect the concern with the existing barriers in

New York State—as opposed to many other states of the Union—which inhibit the development of continuing care retirement communities in this state. The many recommendations brought forth by the conference participants are a clear indication that this long term care alternative is of great interest to potential consumers and providers.

Chapter 10

Programmatic and Operational Issues of Continuing Care Retirement Communities

Daniel Sambol
Craig Duncan
Melvin Katz

While Continuing Care Retirement Communities (CCRCs) are currently not permitted in the state of New York, this chapter on "Programmatic and Operational Problems" is not a mere philosophical abstraction. Fortunately, the states of Massachusetts, New Jersey and Pennsylvania have had direct experience in establishing and operating CCRCs which they were willing to share with us.

Below is a description of apparent differences between current approaches utilized by the nonprofit sector in New York State in the existing long-term care service system as compared with the proposed establishment of CCRCs.

In New York, the nonprofit sector is geared for the most part to serving a dependent and needy population. Potential CCRC residents appear to represent, by comparison, a wealthy population with high levels of service expectations. This fundamental difference in clientele needs to be examined by voluntary boards of directors in terms of their current mission because it may call for a different philosophy of care.

In New York State, the long-term care system is health-oriented and geared to institutional services in contrast to CCRCs which focus on a residential model, i.e., a home for independent, ambula-

Daniel Sambol, Director, Division on Aging, Federation of Protestant Welfare Agencies, Inc., New York, N.Y. Craig Duncan, Executive Director, James A. Eddy Memorial Geriatric Center, Inc., Troy, N.Y. Melvin Katz, Manager, Caring for the Aging Practice, Peat, Marwick, Mitchell & Co., New York, N.Y.

tory, well elderly, with a health care facility and services available but not emphasized.

The corporate structure of the nonprofit facility, if applied to CCRCs, would have to be reconsidered with respect to its not-for-profit status, the possibility of receiving unrelated business income, and its status as a Medicare-Medicaid provider. The issue of subsidization should also be addressed. Experience with subsidized housing under Section 202 and Section 8 in New York State involves inevitable waiting lists while CCRC's require a different approach.

Even the architectural designs for CCRCs are indicative of their difference from non-profit facilities for the elderly. In fact, the residential aspects of the program are highlighted and the health care services are usually less conspicuous. Admission policies represent another source of difference in approach. And a service package in a CCRC must be sold which means a written contract spelling out the responsibilities and obligations of the sponsor and the residents must be completed.

New York State feels it is a most progressive state and state officials believe it spends the most money for institutional care. Overlooked is the value of appropriate housing for keeping people out of skilled nursing facilities. An example often cited was that of a 300-unit apartment house located in New York City approximately twenty-four miles from its suburban-based sponsor which operated a two-level health care facility on its main campus. During five years, only five apartment house residents were transferred to the main campus, four of those going directly to the skilled nursing facility. Clearly there is room for such a housing-oriented program in the continuum of long term care.

Since the CCRC does not stress health but focuses on a secure residence with many support services, it has important preventive elements which may be currently overlooked by New York State.

While New York State is the only State which prohibits CCRCs, it has been suggested that this prohibition might in the end prove to be valuable since New York State could learn from the experiences of other communities where CCRCs are in operation. Had New York State been first, the CCRC industry might have been overregulated.

When the establishment of CCRCs is under consideration, the following operational and program issues must be examined and addressed.

QUALITY OF LIFE AND FACILITIES

A CCRC is a community that must be promoted and sold. It is not a product that people will generally buy unless they are informed about the services available and their value. The quality of service is critical to the success of CCRCs. People entering them have been accustomed to comfortable living. They will pay substantial entrance fees and expect a high standard of service. Potential customers must be made aware of the package of independent living units combined with social, recreational, and dining facilities as well as other amenities. It must be recognized that these communities cater to independent people with a life style they want to maintain. Food services are a major attraction. Housekeeping and maintenance should be of high quality. It has been the experience that CCRC residents frequently form associations and are often articulate and demanding. Emphasis should be placed on the luxurious, gracious life style that the CCRC is able to offer.

While the sizes of CCRCs vary, they are rarely developed with less than two hundred units plus sixty skilled nursing facility beds. Dining and recreational facilities may range in size from twenty thousand to fifty thousand square feet. The CCRC does not offer an institutional program and is not primarily geared to health care although it is part of the package. Health care services typically include a skilled nursing facility, outpatient clinic, and home health and home care services.

CCRC facilities are not rented to outsiders for extra income; they are usually open to residents and their guests but not to the public. Many retain the atmosphere of private clubs. Opening a facility to outsiders not only changes this ambiance but opens the CCRC to the jurisdiction of another city or state department.

There is a view abroad that CCRC residents do not like to have young people around. However, this varies from community to community. Some CCRCs allow young people to visit only; others, such as those in Indiana, have sold pieces of CCRC property for use by younger people because older people have enjoyed their proximity.

One developer reported that he had developed CCRCs in six states (Pennsylvania, Massachusetts, Illinois, Florida, California, Maryland) and had no difficulty in securing certificates of need in any one. It was noted that the New Jersey Department of Health is working on an exclusion in its Certificate of Need (CON) process. It will permit a skilled nursing facility in a CCRC as long as the Skilled Nursing Facility (SNF) is opened to the general public at the outset. In time, as the community's residents require SNF services, they will get priority.

FINANCIAL ISSUES

Financial feasibility in regard to service provision is a critical and delicate area. To achieve success, developers must try to keep the fee low yet provide a high quality level of care. Adequate reserves are essential to assure a sound financial structure so that obvious and concealed costs can be covered. The financial package usually consists of an up-front investment by the residents plus maintenance fee. The contract spells out specifically the services provided and their costs. Such a contract has the advantage of permitting individuals to budget properly since the residents know what their living expenses will be. Even though the contract is not a real estate transaction, New York State and other states treat it like one and require a prospectus which must include a listing of all possible risks.

Feasibility reports are essential though experience has shown that sponsors dislike spending money for them. They can provide realistic numbers and realistic projections. However, individuals are generally not interviewed for these studies since this is not the general practice of accounting firms.

In New York State, the pattern has been to establish feasibility of housing and other developments through market research which does include interviews. The market is then tested in accordance with the Attorney General's office requirements to indicate that the descriptive material is not to be construed as an "offering" but is merely to seek "expressions of interest." At the time a deposit is taken, a prospectus is issued which provides full disclosures. Subsequently, construction is initiated and the residents occupy the facility. Usually, actuaries are not involved in this process.

It is clear that there is a need to understand the market. One cannot make assumptions about the older people who are targeted. A format must be developed to reach that market and the means must be acquired to find the potential customers in a large area.

CCRC sponsors are in a business and need to develop income and build reserves. It has been noted that fifty percent of all new businesses fail. The experience of CCRCs has been far more positive.

However, there are no guarantees of success. Failures need to be examined because important lessons can be learned from them.

There have been some systematic evaluations of existing CCRCs to determine factors which have contributed to successes or failures. The experience in the Philadelphia area as reported in the University of Pennsylvania study indicates that twenty-three successful CCRCs have been established and only two or three are confronting difficulties.

PROMOTIONAL ASPECTS

Another operational issue concerns how one goes about deciding the level of pre-sales at which one can determine the starting date of construction. There is no single answer to that question. It is the sponsor's decision and he may decide to move when ready. In Chicago, one developer waited three years for a specific ratio of pre-sales. Some early applicants died after pre-sales were initiated and the community still is not open. Another agency required a 50 percent pre-sale before starting construction, a process that took two years. In another instance, a lender provided a substantial loan without a single pre-sale because he was convinced that the market study assured success. One developer believed that it took one and a half years to finalize a single sale.

With respect to the variety of units offered, there was a study which found that, of twenty-three subsidized housing developments in Massachusetts in which an effort was made to determine the size of apartment that people wanted, without a single exception, the response was that one-bedroom apartments were preferred over efficiencies. Respondents indicated they needed space and wanted to be able to control their living space. However, it is believed that design has much to do with success. A studio may be very desirable if properly designed.

How is it possible to predict word of mouth influence? People who are satisfied may recommend the community to friends but, if unhappy, may bad-mouth the facility and prevent people from buying in. There seems to be no way to prevent this from happening. Thus a high quality of service is the surest way to promote good recommendations and prevent bad ones. Unlike nursing homes, people who buy into CCRCs are doing so voluntarily.

A major attraction of CCRCs to couples is continuity of care. In those instances where a husband and wife share an apartment and the ill spouse must transfer to the SNF, the well spouse may remain in the apartment nearby, without any additional charge to the couple for the nursing home admission.

Another attraction is the fact that after people enter the community and if they find themselves confronted by financial difficulties, and if the community is well-run, they will not be forced to leave. A well-run community usually sets aside a reserve fund to subsidize such needy individuals. A strong fiscal base probably can be assured through the proper selection of applicants and may minimize the need for subsidization.

In one community, residents are periodically re-qualified financially because sometimes their families take the older person's assets. In these instances a program of financial counseling can prove extremely helpful to the residents.

OTHER CONCERNS

The issue of possible abuse is one that must be addressed. CCRCs require substantial entry fees as an initial investment plus monthly maintenance fees. One way of increasing income is to increase the "turnover" of residents. Encouraging turnover through disincentives to care, that is, allowing deterioration of maintenance and poor quality of care, may lower morale and result in premature death. This deliberate policy certainly is abusive.

One way to prevent such an occurrence is to refund entry fees totally if people wish to leave. By prohibiting an insurance-reserve factor, New York State regulations provide no incentive to individuals to preserve their assets. Neither is there any incentive to the operator to contain expenses. The insurance factor in CCRCs encourages individuals to save and use their funds for themselves.

There has been some concern about the number of people in the housing component who will not use the health component and whether it is appropriate for them to subsidize those who use health services. It is often the case that many residents are willing to pay for the security that the health services are readily available but who hope they will never need them.

Some continuing care communities provide only home health care services instead of needed SNF services, and others cut recreation activities and other amenities in order to contain costs. While it costs less to help an individual remain in his residence than to transfer him to a SNF bed, most communities try to provide the bed if needed. Rarely will activities be cut.

Some program aspects vary from community to community. For example, some communities prohibit the use of alcohol, especially if they are sponsored by religious groups; some discourage a single male from living with a single female, and some do not permit residents to retain their pets. As noted, these policies are highly variable.

SUMMARY

In summary, the typical community is located on a common campus with a package of housing, recreational and health services. Life care implies health care in case of subsequent deterioration. Continuing care implies availability of health care without placing undue stress on it. People do not want to think about it other than to be aware of its availability—a very important concept. Residents usually want to know that an SNF is available so that they can visit their friends and neighbors and be visited, if necessary, in turn.

There seems to be some concensus that CCRCs offer valuable services to a significant sector of the elderly population and should be explored as an option for New York State.

Chapter 11

Financial and Actuarial Steps Recommended for the Development of a Continuing Care Retirement Community in New York State

Alwyn V. Powell
Aaron M. Rose
William B. Sims

This paper will examine issues related to the planning and development of a continuing care retirement community and recommend a step-by-step approach. Actuarial problems will also be explored.

When planning to establish a new continuing care retirement community, the planning process should begin with choosing an appropriate location for the community. After the site has been selected, a preliminary market feasibility study is required to determine whether there is a market for the community. If the market feasibility study indicates a strong probability of success, the next step is to choose a project development team. It is thought that the project should *not* be developed by a committee. Instead, a leader is needed to coordinate the activities of the other members of a development team. This team should include an architect, a marketing consultant, a feasibility consultant, a legal counsel, and a financial consultant. Members of the team are expected to have intermittent involvement in various phases of the community's development which may last from one to two years.

After formation of the project development team, one of the first tasks for the Board of Directors is to address several issues such as:

Alwyn V. Powell, President, A.V. Powell & Associates, Inc., Atlanta, Ga. Aaron M. Rose, C.P.A., Laventhol & Horwath, Philadelphia, Pa. William B. Sims, President, Herbert J. Sims & Co., Inc., New York, N.Y.

(1) what size should the community be? It is believed that a community should have at least 175 independent living units to be economically viable; (2) what type of facilities should be included on the campus? (3) should high-rise or low-rise apartments be built? (4) what is the socio-economic status of the target market? (5) what type of contract provisions should be offered? (6) how long will death and withdrawal refunds last? (7) will an extended health care guarantee be offered that covers the resident for his entire lifetime in the facility, or will the guarantee be limited to a year or less so that those residents who need more utilization pay their own way? (8) will a fully refundable entry fee be offered that could be used to finance a portion of health care costs if a resident permanently transfers to a nursing facility?

After these "product design" policies have been set, the community is ready to consider financing mechanisms. Some of the options are tax-exempt bonds, taxable bonds, government supported program, and conventional mortgages. Financing is a critical area in the development of a community since the community cannot be completed without financing.

From the vantage point of the investment banker, eight issues have to be considered in the development of a project. The first issue concerns the sponsor and his commitment to the organization. The investment banker should determine whether the sponsor has a long-term commitment or is planning to leave the project as soon as construction has been completed. The second issue, relating to product design, is whether there should be a nursing home on site. There is some disagreement on whether it is important for the nursing home to be on the premises. Some believe that it is necessary only to make nursing care available and close enough so that residents have relatively easy access to the facility. Others stress the importance of an on-site nursing facility, however it should not be a prominent feature of the overall architectural design.

A third issue is competition. What is the existing and potential competition in the area? How are other facilities doing? If they are not successful (e.g., low occupancy), is it advisable to add another community in that area?

The fourth issue is market penetration. The investment banker will review the location and take into consideration any natural boundaries, such as a river or highway, that might deter target people from actually moving into the community.

Financial feasibility is a fifth issue. What types and amounts of reserves should the community hold? The feasibility analysis should include sensitivity to financial and actuarial assumptions since no one can predict the future with certainty. The sensitivity analysis allows you to determine whether the community is viable if the expected assumptions do not occur. The feasibility analysis should be performed by a nationally recognized consultant with health care experience.

A sixth issue is presales of apartment units. One rule-of-thumb is a presale rate of 50%. This means that the investment banker typically does not consider financing unless the community has presold 50% of its units with potential entrants paying 10% or more of the initial entry fee. The presale objective, if obtained, gives a strong indication of the success of the community. Although the 50% goal may seem high prior to actual construction, it is generally felt by the investment industry that it is better to stop development and absorb losses before floating a $15 to $20 million bond issue. Inadequate presales may suggest difficulties in achieving full occupancy.

The seventh concern is the caliber of management. Who is going to manage the community after its opening?

The eighth issue concerns the contract design with regard to the kinds of services that will be included with the basic fees as well as those available for an additional charge. Is there in the contract a health care guarantee, of what type and how will such a guarantee be funded? Is there in the contract the entry fee refund provision including when and how much will be refunded?

From the vantage point of an actuary, it can be stated that continuing care appears to be a cost efficient delivery system from a utilization perspective for providing long-term care to the elderly. The "traditional" continuing care concept, where fees do not vary according to residential status (apartment versus nursing care) of the resident, is affordable by a much larger percentage of the potential market than is currently being served by their industry. This percentage is probably not less than 10% and may be as large as 25% or more of the elderly population.

The major actuarial problem concerns funding health care guarantees. The two extremes are referred to as fee-for-service and risk pooling. Under a fee-for-service arrangement, the resident pays for services as they are utilized on an individual basis. In other words, fees change as the resident's residential status changes. Consider for example, an apartment resident who paid $750 per month while living in his/her apartment. After permanent transfer to the nursing home, (s)he would then pay $2,000 per month. Under a risk pooling arrangement, that resident would continue to pay $750 per month after transfer since all residents share on a group basis the costs of health care utilization. Using the risk pooling approach, a resident pays the same fees regardless of his residential status. A variation on this concept is referred to as a limited guarantee where the contract reverts to a fee-for-service arrangement after a fixed number of days in a nursing home.

Currently, there is no dominant trend among *new* starts regarding preference for "fee for service" as opposed to "risk pooling." However, it is interesting to note that several communities which started with extensive guarantees are switching to limited guarantees to restrict their health care liabilities. One of the more important findings of the Wharton School study described by Winklevoss and Powell (1984) was that the "traditional" extensive guarantee is financially viable even with the small populations typically found in retirement communities. However, this assumes that management has utilized proper planning and forecasting procedures using sophisticated management techniques such as those suggested in the book summarizing the Wharton School study. (See Chapter 4 of this volume.)

An advantage of the risk pooling approach is that it provides access to the financial security offered by continuing care to a significant portion of the elderly. Correlatively, a disadvantage of the fee-for-service approach is the restricted potential market due to higher admission rate requirements. It should be noted that the Wharton School study found no case where a resident was ever required to leave a facility if his/her financial resources were depleted for reasons beyond his/her control. The implication of this observation is that whatever type of guarantee is offered, communities appear to adhere to a moral position to always care for their residents. The appeal of fee-for-service contracts is that the community minimizes its financial risks with regard to the liabilities associated with providing long-term care for residents.

Some issues regarding the actuarial/reserve component of regulation are: how is insolvency defined? Is it sufficient to generate sufficient cash flows and meet debt service or should the community be required to actuarially fund 100% of all health care liabilities? What are the objectives of regulation? Does one simply want to protect residents and assets of investors or does one want it to serve as an early warning mechanism? Should regulation be used as a method for standardizing contracts by requiring specific refund provisions and other options? Can regulation be used to define specific pricing methodologies and structures?

The answers to these questions are philosophical and will vary for each state's legislation. However, one suggestion which is in agreement with Winklevoss and Powell (1984) is that whatever form of legislation is developed by New York State, it should include a provision that requires communities to systematically collect and maintain actuarial statistics regarding residents' deaths (mortality) and movements among various levels of care (morbidity). This element is essential for developing a reasonable data base for evaluating a CCRCs financial status.

Chapter 12

Legal Barriers in New York State and Recommendations on How to Deal With Them

James Sanderson
Garrett Heher

The following is a condensed report of a workshop during the course of which several legal issues were addressed that constitute barriers to the development of continuing care communities in the state of New York. Continuing care is defined for this paper as independent living with a health care component; not a priority admission into a health care facility but a continuing care agreement providing health care.

Below are listed all the impediments that are barriers in New York State to the development of life care communities as previously recounted in the chapters by Warner (Chapter 7), Plummer (Chapter 8) and Nurick (Chapter 9); (1) Health Department regulations include two items which have had a chilling effect on continuing care in New York, namely Regulation #414.16 and the Certificate of Need (C.O.N.) process for which New York stipulates very strict requirements; (2) Department of Social Service regulations also prevent continuing care contracts from being written; (3) insurance law also prevents continuing care. It is not possible to mention all the sections, but it is possible that continuing care is subject to the insurance law because it offers a contract for health care in the future or because there is a risk-sharing arrangement. Probably, the insurance department will have to be involved as one of the regulators; (4) the Attorney General's Office considers Continuing Care

James Sanderson, Esq., Tobin & Dempf, Albany, N.Y. Garrett Heher, Esq., Smith, Stratton, Wise, Heher, Brennan, Princeton, N.J.

137

as an offering, a syndication and as such a community would be subject to filing with them; (5) the Division of Housing would also have to be involved in regulation.

OPTIONS AVAILABLE IN NEW YORK STATE

1. One can file an application now to develop a continuing care community as Cohen suggested and try to tough it out. That application will go sideways and get knocked backwards because of so many of the impediments listed above that are going to come into play. The application probably will move through the system eventually but by that time continuing care will be a thing of the past and something new will come up.

2. Another approach is to try to change the regulations, and for this reason contact should be made with the Governor's office. Trying to develop continuing care communities is bound up in so many departments, and so tied into the bureaucratic morass in New York State that it is advisable to have directions for change come from above. One should work through the Governor's office or somewhere close to that level because there are so many departments involved when it comes to changing regulations. The following process might work in New York: file an application which sets forth a proposal from somebody who is planning to develop a continuing care community. The developer is going to raise the crucial issues in the process such as (a) actuarial assumptions, (b) finances and reserves, (c) operation and (d) management. This application will be subject to the Certificate of Need process because part of the application must mention need for health care beds. Probably the facility will have to promise never to make the facility eligible for Medicaid. That does not mean that the residents cannot leave the facility and become eligible for Medicaid. It means that the facility will not be a Medicaid facility with the major implication that the facility will be entirely dependent on private pay. This may not be a good concept but it is one way to get around the problem of how to build additional health care beds in New York which will be needed if the continuing care community is going to be true to the concept of continuing care.

What sort of model legislation should be drawn up? James Sanderson and Garrett Heher were instrumental in writing the Model Act for Continuing Care for the American Association of Homes for the Aging (1980). The Act takes a limited regulatory oversight position and it is a disclosure act. It does not require reserves; it does not review nor approve the actuarial assumptions. It probably requires very little of what ought to be required. Thus, the potential consumer must be made fully aware of all the ramifications and all the financial angles before he can make an intelligent choice to buy into such a community.

In New Jersey there does not seem to be any difficulty in protecting both the consumer and provider. Gary Heher has a client, Presbyterian Homes of New Jersey, which owns six homes only one of which provides continuing care and only one of which, therefore, serves people from the middle and upper income brackets. All the other facilities involve extensive, if not complete, subsidy in one form or another but they are every bit as nice as the continuing care facility.

From a practical standpoint, the market situation should also be considered. It does not make much sense to prohibit continuing care because this means taking this option away from people and forcing people who wish this option out of state. Many people apply to the Presbyterian Homes in New Jersey who live in New York. A gentleman from Rochester, N.Y. told about somebody who unwillingly moved from Rochester, where he wanted to stay after retiring to the community of Foulkeways in Gwynned, Pennsylvania because there were no continuing care communities in New York. If this option is made available and if the market is there, New Yorkers would soon be taking advantage of it. The lack of availability of this option not only seems unfair to those who wish it but seems a wrong economic decision if one looks at the dollars that are generated. For example, one home which has expenses of $8 million dollars pays $356,000, for local property taxes. New York seems to be denying itself that opportunity.

There may be a question about advertising and marketing practices used by continuing care communities which are located in other states. New York State law requires truth in advertising. This law requires registering of any real estate offering even if it is located in New Jersey. Thus it has been determined that Presbyterian Homes of New Jersey are not exempt from this New York law however they are exempt from a similar law in New Jersey because there is neither a sale nor a lease involved. Presbyterian Homes has been complying with this New York statute. The statute requires registration, much like the American Association of Homes for the

Aging Model Act does. This process is very time consuming and expensive and requires giving many details in the form of prospectuses to be available both to each individual as well as to New York State.

Given all of the legal impediments in New York State it is estimated that it will probably take several years before there will be an operative continuing care retirement community. It is intended that this volume and the conference on which it is based will speed up the process. There will be an on-going follow-up process instituted whereby the contributors to this volume can keep abreast of any progress made in New York State.*

---

*Editor's Note. On October 26, 1984, the American Association of Homes for the Aged announced its development of a national accreditation program for continuing care retirement communities with the support of a grant awarded by the Pew Memorial Trust. The primary goals of AAHA's new accreditation program are to educate the public about all aspects of continuing care retirement communities and to ensure the continuation of high quality administration and services as the continuing care field expands. AAHA's program will involve establishing standards of excellence to govern the administration and operation of continuing care retirement communities; developing an application, review and assessment process for accreditation status; and conducting a national public education campaign. For further information about this program, contact AAHA, 1050 17th Street, NW, Suite 770, Washington, DC 20036. AAHA is also in the process of compiling a summary of existing statutes regulating continuing care retirement communities, currently in effect in the various states.

Chapter 13

New York State Public Policy Barriers, Changes Needed and Recommendations for Action

Erika Teutsch
Abraham Monk
Laurence Lane
Marcia Steinhauer

The purpose of this chapter is to raise questions and make recommendations concerning the potential development of continuing care retirement communities in New York State. An attempt is also made to determine whether existing policies and regulations, which in effect prohibit most models of continuing care retirement communities, should be changed and if so how. The discussion will focus on four issues: the need (or market) for such communities, the nature and the locus of regulation and the problem of a two-tier system.

1. Should the door be opened in New York State to the development of Continuing Care Retirement Communities? Is there a real need and a market in New York State? It is known that CCRCs exist in other states, although not yet in very large numbers. Furthermore, it is also known that those that exist have very long waiting lists. Is the existing law forcing New Yorkers to move to other states if they wish to avail themselves of this option? What kind of numbers are being speculated about? Does current state policy, in fact, encourage circumvention of existing regulations? Has the develop-

Erika Teutsch, Metropolitan Area Coordinator for Adult Services, NYS Dept. for Social Services, New York, N.Y. Abraham Monk, Director, Brookdale Institute on Aging and Adult Human Development, Columbia University, New York, N.Y. Laurence Lane, Director for Non-Proprietary and Special Programs, American Health Care Association, Washington, D.C. Marcia B. Steinhauer, Assistant Chair and Associate Professor, Graduate Program for Administrators, Rider College, Laurenceville, N.J.

141

ment of retirement communities and programs encouraged developers to get around the existing state prohibitions and thus operate without any control from state agencies because the system encourages that circumvention? Why has there not been any great pressure on state agencies for a change in policy? State agencies have not heard from the consumer advocacy groups, from AARP, from AHAB, or from other organizations that represent the elderly. Is there a reason why the consumer advocates have not come to the state to say "open up the doors, we really want this?" Is it just a developer's dream to create new models and not a program that the elderly really need? The answers to any of these questions are yet to be determined and there is the need to explore them before development of such communities is encouraged.

2. If the door is to be opened to CCRCs, there is a consensus repeated throughout this volume that their development would have to be accompanied by some regulation. New York State's history, philosophy and political climate almost mandate that any basic program of this nature would require some state oversight and some state regulation. The potential for fraud, by just leaving it to the free market, is there as is known from experience with the nursing home scandals. There are also by-products and the problems created for the poor and the middle income market when the real estate industry housing developers are left to their own devices. In this instance, should the elderly be considered a vulnerable population that by definition, needs state intervention and protection?

3. What is it that needs to be regulated? Who is to regulate? The areas that need to be considered include certification and accreditation both of the operators and of the program; the whole range of financial regulations including financial disclosure of a reserve fund, setting up of escrow provisions; setting up provisions in case of bankruptcy; considering third party involvement in the financing as well as the regulation of these communities. Should there be model provider-resident agreements that have to be approved by some state agency? What about the Medicaid eligibility of residents in these communities? Should resident councils be mandated? How should residents' rights be protected? Should advertising and prospectus information be regulated? The answer to the question of who is to regulate depend, of course, on what is regulated. If the focus is on the financial piece of these programs and communities, we would want to look to the Insurance Department, the Housing Finance Agency, or the Banking Department for regulation. If the

main focus is on the service aspect of the communities, then we are talking about the Office for the Aging, Social Services, Health, or perhaps a new agency. There are many possibilities and combinations of possibilities. One recommendation is that, perhaps instead of developing a model demonstration project, (as is sometimes done when new service concepts are created), the matter should be approached from the opposite end by encouraging the state agencies to develop a model regulatory system with a clear lead agency before encouraging programs to develop and apply.

4. Will a two tier service model be encouraged by permitting the development of these communities? CCRCs appear to be almost exclusively for middle and upper income groups and by definition we will be forcing lower income and poor people into the nursing homes. Will we end up with retirement communities for the middle class and nursing homes filled with poor people only because they will not have the financial resources to invest in these communities? What is the state's role in preventing such a situation? At least, the state should determine if this model can be adapted to include people in the lower income groups?

A major question is: what is the next step to take in order to maintain the momentum, to expedite mechanisms and to pursue some of the open ends? Two documented facts seem to support the argument for development of CCRCs in or out of this state: (1) the new census data shows that three years have been added to the American life span within a single decade; and (2) the multiple disabilities that are associated with increased age. The combination of these phenomena requires a residential setting that provides for complete independence while offering a full range of services. Moreover, these services should be calibrated to the changing needs of the individual. There seems to be every reason to include CCRCs among the range of innovative ways of coping with the dual desires of older persons for both independence and security. Now is the time to look for models to determine which one should be adopted, to promote interest in developing regulatory models and to encourage interest in the people who need to be involved in this process.

RECOMMENDATIONS FOR ACTION

1. New York State should be encouraged to get something started as state action, whether it be legislative or regulatory and to begin to move towards relaxing some specific restrictions. It is

recommended that New York State's government move to make some appropriate changes, or study which changes are, in fact, appropriate at this time.

2. New regulations should be built on what already exists and explore how that can be expanded and extended. There are programs and models in New York State that can be built on. This may be the most constructive way to proceed, in terms of both the development and regulation of these programs. The result would probably be an option similar to some kinds of continuing care community found in other states.

3. More input from potential consumers should be elicited to find out what is really needed. Since existing experience in other states is very limited, New York State residents need to indicate what it is they want and need.

4. There should be an opportunity within the State of New York to develop the CCRC concept. Public and consumer education should include explanations of the concept of CCRC as being not just a nursing home and should emphasize to older individuals the importance of entering a CCRC while they are still active.

5. It should be recognized that the health care component is but one aspect of the total CCRC concept. This notion should be put in the proper perspective by the health bureaucracy in its oversight activities of CCRCs.

6. There should be legislation drafted and enacted to assure that financial resources of CCRCs are secure against their possible failure.

7. CCRCs should include the potential utilization of insurance policies as part of the entrance fees to stabilize financial feasibility.

8. The Consumer Protection Board should be a focal point within the state for protecting the future of the elderly. This Board should have early involvement in the development of CCRCs.

9. It is suggested that Columbia University might codify those regulations that apply to the area of continuing care regulation beyond the applicable statutes in the Departments of Social Services, and Health. Codification is needed of tax issues, tax exemption questions, and certificate of need. This probably should be done before approaching legislators.

In conclusion, it seems fair to say that there certainly is an interest at the state level to begin to open the doors to CCRCs. However, the state needs to hear a great deal more both from the potential consumers and from those providers in the field who are now operating related facilities. Many of these persons know from their own experience what the needs are and what modifications the present system might need to be able to offer some kinds of continuing care options. Such can be defined in a variety of ways. It is recommended that a summary report and the proceedings in this volume should be directed not only to state officials and public policy makers, but also to the current providers of related services and to those groups that represent the potential consumers. It is, after all, they who should do some more thinking about whether continuing care communities are needed in New York State.

PART VI:
EXECUTIVE SUMMARY

The following is a portion of the Executive Summary which was sent to the Governor of the State of New York, to policy makers and persons concerned with the issues of retirement communities in New York State. The response on the part of state officials was positive and the issues are receiving increased attention at the state and local levels.

While this is a summary of the conference presentations, workshop reports and recommendations as they were presented to the Plenary Sessions, it essentially captures the spirit of the book and it is for this reason that we have chosen to include it in this volume.

THE CONFERENCE PROGRAM

Addresses

Welcome	Barry Gurland, M.D., Director, Center for Geriatrics & Gerontology, Columbia University
Prologue and Introduction	Ian A. Morrison, Ed.D., President, Greer-Woodycrest Children's Services
Policies on Retirement Communities in New York State: Historical Background and Current Status	George Warner, M.D., Special Advisor, NYS Department of Health, and Corinne Plummer, Deputy Commissioner, NYS Department of Social Services

Addresses continued

Ethical Issues in Continuing Care	Msgr. Charles J. Fahey, Director, Third Age Center, Fordham University
Legal Regulation of the Continuing Care Retirement Community Industry	David L. Cohen, Esq., Ballard, Spahr, Andrews & Ingersoll
Continuing Care Retirement Communities: Issues in Financial Management	Howard E. Winklevoss, Ph.D., President, Winklevoss & Associates, Inc.
A Short History of Management Organization, Models, Processing Methods, and Problems to Worry About in a For-Profit Life Care Community	Frank E. Elliott, Founder, Pine Run Community, and Chairman of the Board, Life Care Society of America, Inc.
Continuing Care—Consumer Choice: from Compact to Contracts	Laurence F. Lane, President, Laurence F. Lane Associates
Political and Social Implications of Continuing Care Contracts for New York State	Lloyd Nurick, Executive Director, New York State Association of Homes for the Aged

Workshops

A. Public Policy Issues	Chairman: Abraham Monk, Ph.D., Director, Brookdale Institute on Aging and Adult Development, Columbia University
B. Legal Issues and Barriers	Chairman: James Sanderson, Esq., American Association of Homes for the Aging, Member of House of Delegates
C. Financial and Actuarial Aspects	Chairman: Aaron Rose, CPA, Partner, Laventhol and Horwath, Philadelphia

Workshops continued

D. Programmatic and
   Operational Problems

Chairman: Craig A. Duncan,
Executive Director, James A.
Eddy Memorial Fund

E. Consumer Interests

Chairman: Patricia Cook,
Member of the Board, Loretto
Geriatric Center, Syracuse,
New York

SUMMARY OF PRESENTATIONS

Policies on Retirement Communities in New York State: Historical Background and Current Status

Explaining current policy affecting life care communities (or facilities similar to them) were *George Warner, M.D.*, Special Advisor, NYS Dept. of Health, and *Corinne Plummer,* Deputy Commissioner, NYS Dept. of Social Services.

Dr. Warner traced the events which led to the present prohibition of life care contracts, beginning with the appointment of the Folsom Committee by Governor Rockefeller in 1964. Charged to study the escalating costs of hospital care, the committee a year and a half later turned in a report on nine major problem areas. Subsequent study and action resulted in Article XXVIII of the Public Health Law—Article XXVIII utilizing the word "hospital" in a very broad context to embrace a variety of providers at many different levels.

The provision within Article XXVIII of greatest concern to this Conference is that which says that facilities to be constructed, or facilities intending to add beds, renovate or change ownership, must meet several tests in order to secure approval for same at the State level: a Certificate of Need/Resource Control Test; a Character Competence Test; and of greatest interest to this Conference, a Financial Feasibility test—evidence that the planned project could meet financial demands now *and in the future.* Anticipated future sources of revenue had to be sufficient to meet operating costs. The State could not be viewed as a bail-out entity if a project's resources were not equal to the financial requirements, especially if the residents' own personal resources were to run dry.

With concern for financial feasibility the reason, the provision now in effect that indirectly blocks continuing care retirement communities in New York State is the one stating "the operator shall not enter into any contract or agreement with a patient, resident, next of kin and/or sponsor for life care of the patient or resident." The concern behind this provision seemed justified when the New York State Association of Homes for the Aged reported in meetings that some members were beginning to suffer from the financial threat of life care contracts which their endowments and aid from other sources could no longer sustain.

Thus there is now in effect in NY State the original provision which prohibits advance payments for more than three months at a time. Since these code requirements went into effect, in February of 1966, the State has seen "no reasons to change prohibition against life-care contracts in the *health care aspect of the long-term care spectrum.*" Furthermore, in view of signs of further increasing costs of SNF and HRF care, retaining "these prohibitions against . . . financial arrangements that may, in fact, become disastrous to sponsoring institutions, does seem to make great sense."

Elaborating further on Dr. Warner's presentation of the role of State agencies in the history and provision of life care services, Deputy Commissioner Plummer made the point "that New York State has yet to address continuing care, particularly the concept of continuing care communities, as a distinct entity. . ." However, issues relating to continuing care, such as life care contracts, have "had a persistent and somewhat problematic place in a number of State programs." The reality is a kind of "piecemeal" response.

Various laws and departments impose conditions and set standards for services that would be included in the delivery of continuing care. But, "despite this extensive involvement in most of the individual elements of continuing care—consideration of promotion of continuing care retirement communities, of coordinated oversight, or of the role of public funding in such settings has been limited, and mostly negative."

Ms. Plummer went on to recount the history of life care and the contracts for such care in residential facilities, noting that nonprofit organizations, frequently church related, have been responding to the needs of the aged for some time, some of them becoming very sophisticated. Initially, the Board of Social Welfare had oversight responsibilities for such facilities, but regulatory changes occurred with Article XXVIII, as well as with the introduction of Medicare and Medicaid in the late 60s.

Subsequent reclassification led to some facilities closing, some being designated as homes for the aged under the supervision of the Department of Social Services and the Board of Social Welfare, and others being classified as nursing facilities under the supervision of the Health Department. This reclassification affected a number of organizations which offered life care contracts. While initial planning and regulation intended joint supervision by Health and the Board, so that adult homes could maintain infirmaries, that joint effort was never realized.

Reclassification and transfers of supervision did lead to "interesting problems"—such as the level of care issue. What kind of facility could be certified for what kind of care? What would happen to individual residents and the financial viability of a facility if regulatory oversight demanded abrupt closure?

The State did, in 1977, actively discourage life care agreements in adult homes, since it felt that persons requiring a particular degree of skilled nursing care ought not to be retained in a facility not equipped to provide it, a facility served by a social services staff rather than a health services staff.

Yet another factor complicating the viability of life care contracts was the set of regulations concerning eligibility for life care under Medicaid—when an individual's or a facility's resources were depleted.

In closing, Ms. Plummer acknowledged that

> It may appear that *all* current policies impacting continuing care retirement communities run counter to the interests of many of you at this conference. It is, instead, I think, an appropriate threshold for carefully examining the place of these communities and the type and degree of government involvement warranted. Consumer protection, level of care, joint oversight, State regulation and other important issues will be explored in depth in the discussion sessions. The results should help New York look closely at the potential role of Continuing Care Retirement Communities in this State.

Ethical Issues in Continuing Care

Speaking to the full assembly of conference participants, *Msgr. Charles J. Fahey,* director of the Third Age Center at Fordham University, set forth an "ethical framework" within which conferees could assess the appropriateness of New York State's current prohibition against continuing care communities.

Msgr. Fahey identified three key groups that would be affected by new public policy, groups whose legitimate interests must therefore be considered in any discussion of that public policy. They are the potential user, the provider of services and society in general.

Msgr. Fahey noted that among potential users, evidence indicates that there is a growing interest in continuing care communities and that the principal attraction of continuing care communities to such persons is the sense of security which these facilities offer. However, Msgr. Fahey cautioned that while continuing care communities seem to be a reasonable option for a large number of persons, these communities should not be considered the best option for all individuals. Indeed, he noted that the sense of security and community-living inherent in continuing care communities may for some persons create a dependency which in turn may lead to a "process of withdrawal."

Because the buyer of continuing care services will, through the natural process of aging, become increasingly vulnerable, the seller (or provider of services) has a unique responsibility to the buyer. And Msgr. Fahey outlined several ethical issues which the seller must address before offering continuing care services to a potential user. For instance, the seller must decide what specific services will be offered to the buyer; what will happen if the buyer is no longer able to pay for these services; how potential conflicts between the buyer and the seller will be resolved; and what assurances can he, the seller, offer in terms of his ability to continue to provide services over an extended period of time. Failure to resolve these issues, Msgr. Fahey warned, has historically led to "tragic examples of poor planning and unethical practices."

In the light of a growing interest in continuing care communities and as New York State, representing society in general, prepares to reconsider its public policy, Msgr. Fahey urged conferees to examine several key issues.

— Has the state of the art of actuarial projections developed sufficiently to assure buyer/seller that future needs can be met?
— Are there sufficient regulatory models from other states which New York State could use as guidelines?
— If New York does allow continuing care communities to operate within the State, should such facilities have nursing homes?

And if so, could these facilities sustain themselves financially?
— Finally, if regulations permit changes in original agreements, would changing circumstances lead to two levels of care: one for the affluent and one for the poor?

Msgr. Fahey called upon conferees to address these questions during the course of the conference and in so doing to discern those values and facts which will provide an ethical basis for State policy.

Legal Regulations of the Continuing Care Retirement Community Industry

David L. Cohen, an attorney with Ballard, Spahr, Andrews & Ingersoll, provided conference participants with an overview of the present regulatory environment around the country, discussed his concerns about the state of New York's current law, and explained why he believes regulation of continuing care communities is important for both the industry and the people it serves.

According to Cohen, there are three regulatory approaches currently in practice in the United States. The first is comprehensive statutory legislation which includes specific types of regulatory provisions. Ten states have taken this approach. The second approach is nonregulation—either because there is no compelling need to create such legislation as in those thirty states which have three or less continuing care retirement communities or because comprehensive statutes are still in the process of being formulated as in New Jersey, Pennsylvania, Ohio and several other states. The third approach is limited regulation of continuing care communities. New York State falls into this category.

Cohen noted that two different interpretations can be applied to New York's current law. The first interpretation holds that New York State's law *intends* to prohibit "life care, continuing care, and anything like life care or continuing care, that is, with an entrance fee up front and a monthly payment." This interpretation, however, would not exclude communities which split residential and health aspects and which finance each through a "pay as you go" policy.

The second interpretation holds that New York State *does not intend* to prohibit "continuing care" but rather "life care" in its pure form. Mr. Cohen defined "life care" as the kind of care which promises complete care for the rest of a person's life for *one set fee,* paid entirely in advance or with one large entrance fee and a set monthly fee. "Continuing care," Cohen explained, differs from "life care" in that the entrance fee is allocated exclusively to capital expenditures and *all basic services are paid for through a monthly fee which can be adjusted for inflation.* Cohen based support of this interpretation on precedent set in Pennsylvania, noting Pennsylvania regulation "worded almost precisely the same as New York's has absolutely no effect in deterring the development of an identical industry. . ." Indeed, Cohen reminded his listeners that Pennsylvania "has the third largest number of continuing care retirement communities in the country." However, Cohen stated that it is his belief that both the consumer and the industry would be best served if New York State got "rid of a regulation which purports to prohibit continuing care and make it clear that we're not going to prohibit the industry, we're going to regulate it to make it safe."

Cohen defended his belief in the need for comprehensive statutes to govern continuing care retirement communities. He noted that good statutory regulations increase certainty in the industry. Clearly defined contractual obligations reduce the potential of costly lawsuits, and adequate reserve requirements increase a facility's certainty of survival. For reasons such as these, Cohen predicted that regulations will eventually be enacted in all states. And he called upon participants to carefully consider how New York State should regulate its continuing care retirement industry warning that "the way your regulation looks will affect very substantially the quality of the industry that develops in your state."

Continuing Care Retirement Communities: Issues in Financial Management

Dr. Howard D. Winklevoss, president of Winklevoss & Associates and a participant in the University of Pennsylvania's comprehensive study of continuing care retirement communities, discussed several critical pitfalls in the financial management of CCRCs.

One of the key problems inherent in the financial management of CCRC's, according to Dr. Winklevoss, "is the very deceptive nature of the income and cash flow of these communities over the first decade and a half." During this time, CCRC's invariably show substantial profits because health care utilization is usually quite low. As a result there is frequently a tendency to "run the finances of the community in such a way that the monies coming in equal the amount going out." When health care utilization does finally mature, the community discovers it has a tremendous unfunded health care liability.

Dr. Winklevoss explained that two factors contribute to this problem. First, generally accepted account principles (GAAP) are not adequate for the task of setting fees to provide reserve funds for long term health care obligations. Second, board members of non-profit CCRCs often lack an understanding of the long term financial commitment, namely, that the health care guarantee is a deferred obligation which must be funded. These board members are therefore disturbed when their community shows what seems to be substantial "profits" during the first ten years, and they are inclined to spend this money on behalf of the residents or to underprice the community—thus depleting the reserve fund.

Another common problem in the financial management of CCRC's, Dr. Winklevoss told his listeners, is the accounting procedure for the earning of entry fees. Indeed, he said, "There are no communities, to my knowledge, that are earning entry fees correctly."

About half of the continuing care retirement communities earn entry fees over residents' life expectancies. However, as Dr. Winklevoss pointed out, half of the persons in a community will live beyond the average life expectancy. Therefore, the CCRC will have earned its income too quickly. About 40% to 50% of the CCRCs recognize this problem. However, even they fail to factor in inflation. Dr. Winklevoss recommended that CCRC's earn the entry fee in very small portions initially and then in ever-increasing amounts while increasing monthly fees at the rate of inflation.

Recognizing that predicting a population's life expectancy and future health care utilization will never be an exact science, Dr. Winklevoss maintained that if pension plans can estimate needed reserves, CCRC's can certainly arrive at credible actuarial estimates which they can continue to track over time. Indeed, he recommended that a certified actuarial review be required in regulations for CCRC's. And he urged CCRC's to develop a national data base of actuarial statistics, noting, "We need to share data as insurance companies do."

Criticizing CCRC's for the tendency *not* to hire professional actuaries, Dr. Winklevoss told his audience, "If these communities are going to work, they have to be run like a business. . . . You had better have professional accountants, you had better have professional lawyers, actuaries and so forth. If you do not want to make these kinds of expenditures, do not get involved with a CCRC. . . . All the good intentions that we have by caring for the aged will not keep these organizations financially sound.''

In concluding, Dr. Winklevoss touched on the topic of regulating the industry. He contended that despite considerable research, ''we do not know enough about the industry.'' He therefore recommended that regulations be legislated on the state level to allow for experimentation rather than attempt to institute federal policy at this time.

A Short History of Management Organization and Models in a Privately Owned Life Care Village at Pine Run, Doylestown, Bucks County, Pennsylvania

Frank E. Elliott, founder and chairman of the board of the Life Care Society of America, chronicled the evolving management style of the Life Care Village at Pine Run since its founding in 1976. He did so in order to illustrate how various forms of managerial organization can be used as tools ''in defining and providing social gerontological support and geriatric health care services to members and patients residing in a life care community.''

Pine Run, Elliott explained, is a privately owned, life care village which serves, at any one time, 525 elderly persons both in good and poor health. It is a fully integrated geriatric, health care station which offers maximum guarantees. The physical plant is composed of 300 terraced apartments in 19 neighborhoods which surround a recreation center and a shopping mall. In addition, Pine Run has a five-storied, 236-bed geriatric rehabilitation ''medical hotel.'' The average age of the residents is 81, and the staff numbers over 250 full-time employees.

Based on the belief ''that the members (Pine Run residents). . . were the experts in what is needed and wanted, and often held the best answer as to how these demands could conveniently and satisfactorily be delivered,'' the management was committed to membership participation in both the formation and ongoing development of managerial policy and strategy. Elliott termed this approach the ''as if'' model—''as if members and patients were founder, manager, and caregiver.''

Pine Run experienced three distinct transitions in managerial organization during the course of its development. During the initial phase of moving in and starting up, Elliott explained, Pine Run management adhered to a "traditional multi-tier, hierarchal organizational format." Pine Run chose this vertical structure for three reasons. First, during ongoing construction of Pine Run, new residents "needed 'quick hands-on' person-to-person management" to handle inevitable crises. Second, this form of management provided a clear sense of stability and order "which assuaged members' psychological need for order." Third, this style of organization, which is "well-known in traditional community voluntary undertakings," helped to build strong member input.

"Once the move-in phase was completed and the community had reached an early stability," Elliott told his listeners, "a new phase of management seemed needed." Pine Run decided to develop an organizational form similar to the multi-national conglomerate, namely, "the techno-bureaucratic hierarchal organization." Mr. Elliott explained that the Pine Run management felt that this structure was the most useful way to organize all operating and program activities for in-depth scrutiny. During this phase, many expensive professional personnel were hired. And it was these professionals, operating as subsidiary companies, who began to gather primary data for storage on a data-based computer system and who established a business atmosphere based on "proof of results."

Once Pine Run was completely computer-based, according to Mr. Elliott, the techno-bureaucratic structure was no longer needed. In its place, management developed a "horizontal synergistic team-based computer-informed organization" which is still in operation today.

This form of managerial organization breaks down into four groups, namely, the core team, the team assembly, the team participants, and the computer as technical executive. The core team is composed of the president and five key executives who supervise funds management, sustaining services, health enrichment, hospitality, and management systems, respectively. The team assembly consists of thirty program managers who are responsible for programs such as estate planning, maintenance, food services, occupational therapy, etc. Members and patients comprise the team participants. Two members of the elected Villager governing body audit monthly meetings of both the core team and the team assembly. Mr. Elliott noted that these team participants have been "especially helpful in key policy-making areas." Finally, the computer as technical executive gathers data on Pine Run business activities as well as medical, social, biographic, psychological and financial data on all members and patients. Based on this data, Pine Run maintains business plans for each program which include "a market demand plan, capital expenditures plan, cash management plan and a projected profit and loss statement and balance sheet for the year, accompanied by a statement of assumptions, business and service objectives, income and expense worksheets." Data-based information also allows management "to catch unacceptable trends and to forecast variants as well as to research program improvement."

Elliott acknowledged that the evolution of Pine Run's organizational format "involved taking some perilous risks." However, he noted: "Management has grown intensively through use of business management discipline, computer technology and open dialogue with those it serves in a dynamic gerontological milieu. . . . The gerontological designs of Pine Run management and facility infrastructure provide Villagers with a special kind of efficiency that makes longitudinal common sense, even for the very, very old."

Continuing Care—Consumer Choice: From Compact to Contracts

In his segment of the conference presentation, *Laurence F. Lane,* president of Laurence F. Lane Associates, sketched the development of formalized, contractual agreements between provider and consumer within continuing care retirement communities.

Lane pointed out that "historically the communal approach to sharing and caring constituted an informal compact among members of the community." He then compared the differences between "Gemeinschaft" (community-based relationships) and "Gesellschaft" (business-based relationships) which were first discussed by 19th century philosophers in the wake of the industrial revolution "to the distinction between community-based service provider mechanism represented by the ideal continuing care community and the contrasting public contract for shelter and services from nursing homes developed as an offshoot of the Federal domestic policies since the 1930's."

Noting that a number of changes "threatened the primary bond of trust which was the basis of informal compacts" traditionally offered by CCRC's, Lane observed that CCRCs were now beginning to incorporate formalized contracts into their relationship with the consumer (or community members). He listed seven key changes which brought about this melding of "Gemeinschaft" and "Gesselschaft" in CCRC's. They are (1) economic uncertainties caused by inflation or recessions; (2) changing demographics such as the declining mortalities; (3) service approach changes from primarily social care to a combination of social and medical care; (4) changing public expectations regarding the level of professionalism in staffing, types of amenities, etc.; (5) changing public requirements such as fire safety codes and minimum wage laws; (6) changing technology in medical care; and (7) changing business approaches in response to long-term service needs which require greater business expertise.

The "formalization of obligation," Lane noted, has run the spectrum "from cryptic admissions agreements to nearly unreadable legal contracts." Indeed, he observed, the provider often has several different contracts to offer a consumer.

Despite the lack of standardized contracts, Lane pinpointed eight general areas which are covered in most CCRC's contracts. They are (1) a definition of services, coverages and accommodations, including hospitalization, transfer to nursing home facilities, a physician's services, registered nursing services, exclusions and areas of non-coverage, and apartment features; (2) a definition of fees, including a statement of both the endowment fee and the monthly fee including provisions for increases in the monthly fee; (3) admissions requirements, including minimum age, minimum level of assets and monthly income, and medical insurance in addition to medicare; (4) stipulations for termination of a contract; (5) conditions which will allow for transfer from an apartment to another accommodation; (6) the refund policy, including probationary entry and refund as well as certain refunds under specified conditions; and (8) a statement of the consumer's right to collective representation.

Noting that contractual rights are "probably only as important as their enforcement," Lane reviewed four approaches to enforcement which are currently in practice. They include (1) legislation embodied in state statutes, the majority of which require state certification of the continuing care provider, full disclosure laws, and financial requirements for escrowing entrance fees during construction and mandating certain audit and lien requirements, and establishing a procedure for addressing conflicts; (2) provider self-policing such as professional accreditation; (3) resident self-governance; and (4) consumer awareness through affirmative disclosure requirements and through policing of misinformation.

In the beginning of his address, Lane raised "the question

whether the formalization of the agreement between the provider and consumer have undermined the communal positive of the continuing care retirement community.'' As he summed up his remarks, Mr. Lane commended the change from informal compacts between the consumer and the provider to contractual agreements, noting that contracts have ensured a balance between the provider and the consumer and that they have further assured the public of the abilities of a provider to meet the consumer's needs.

Political and Social Implications of Continuing Care Contracts for New York State

In seeking to tie together the preceding presentations, *Lloyd Nurick,* executive director of New York State Association of Homes for the Aged, outlined New York State's changing social policy toward continuing care retirement communities in relation to the potential demands such changes will place on future legislation.

Nurick observed that New York State is ''the only state in the union with prohibitions against life care through health care level.'' The reasons for this approach, he contended, have their roots in New York's ''unique structuring of society,'' which Nurick noted, is a society very ''similar to the Western European Welfare State. . . . Our attitudes toward service focus on government regulations and government initiated programming as well as equality of services and equal access to services.'' As a result, ''the concept of selective living arrangements,'' which is typified by CCRCs, ''may be antithetical to the social and political perceptions of New Yorkers.''

Nonetheless, Nurick pointed out, New York is beginning to witness a change in attitude toward CCRCs. Indeed, in the light of new economic circumstances both at the national and state level as well as New York's new emphasis on a strong economic base, New York State is beginning to realize that CCRCs may offer some benefits to the State. Those benefits include additional property and income tax revenues, more jobs for New Yorkers, and a decline in the exodus of New York's elderly middle class.

Practical as well as social changes also have fostered a greater interest in CCRCs according to Nurick. The growth in housing for the elderly, better health and medical care, and the dramatic increase in outreach programs have lessened the need for health-related or domiciliary care facilities. Moreover, Mr. Nurick explained, modern Americans are more independent; they tend to eschew group settings (such as the domiciliary care facility). And as spouses live longer, he speculated, the need for health-related facilities is further postponed. Finally, the image of the nursing home continues to suffer from the scandals of the mid-seventies and is therefore considered the least desirable option by many persons. The cumulative effect of these changes, Mr. Nurick noted, is that "the middle level care of nursing homes is disappearing" while continuing care retirement communities are growing in popularity.

Given the growing drive to establish CCRCs in New York, the State must decide if it wants to regulate this industry. "Some people," Nurick noted, "have suggested you're better off having it (regulation) in law because it protects the consumer, protects the provider, protects the state. Others have said you're better off without laws because we can work within the structure we have and it allows for innovation."

If the State does decide to regulate CCRCs, Nurick observed, it must resolve several questions. A few of these questions are: should one or several agencies be involved in regulating CCRCs? Should certificates of need be required? And should medicaid be prohibited or made available to CCRCs? Nurick warned that "if there is government intervention, at least there must be coordination among agencies in order to allow facilities that are going to be continuing care retirement communities to become functioning organizations without having to go through a series of processes that take years and delay an outcome that is to the benefit of the frail and elderly who cannot wait."

Nurick suggested that New York State allow "only" voluntary sponsorship and operation of CCRCs." And he listed four reasons in support of this view. One, he felt that a community or religious based organization improved a CCRCs potential marketing success. Two, he contended that sponsoring entities would ensure the quality and excellence of care. Three, pointing to evidence based on an analysis of Pennsylvania's CCRCs, he argued that denominational facilities are less likely to develop severe financial problems than developer-oriented facilities. And four, he observed that even when a denominational facility does incur financial problems, as in the case of Pacific Homes, voluntary groups can and have lent their support to the failing facility.

In closing his address, Nurick reviewed four general conclusions from the conference, namely, that CCRCs are feasible in New

York; CCRCs "probably should be tried in New York State;" CCRCs will develop, "one way or the other, with or without legislation"; and finally, that considerable research on CCRCs still needs to be analyzed and discussed before issues affecting the industry can be resolved.

SUMMARIES OF WORKSHOP PRESENTATIONS

Plenary Session

Out of the workshops came a series of reports and recommendations intended to accomplish the goal set forth by Dr. Gurland in his opening remarks.

Workshop A. Public Policy Issues

Recorder: Erika Teutsch,
Metropolitan area coordinator for the Division of Adult Services Activities, NYC Region
NYS Department of Social Services

Recorder Teutsch reported that this panel focused its attention on public policy issues *only with respect to* the potential development in New York State of continuing care retirement communities. It was noted that such communities are currently "pretty much prohibited," given existing state level policies and regulations, although there do exist some models that are fairly close to such communities in other states.

In discussing this topic, the panel realized that the whole subject of public policy issues was too broad and too deep to permit the group to reach firm conclusions. The discussion therefore "focused [on] four basic areas/four basic problems."

Basic Questions—Concerns Raised

1. Should the door be opened in New York State to the development of continuing care retirement communities?

— Is there a real need in New York State—is there a market?
— Are New Yorkers being forced out of their own state for certain types of care? Are there sufficient numbers of them to re-

quire a serious consideration? Do we have sufficient information on this?
— Does current state policy encourage circumvention of existing regulations, and does circumvention in turn make any kind of control impossible?
— Why have we not seen pressure on state agencies to permit this development?
— Why have we not heard from consumer groups, such as AARP?
— Is this really just a developer's dream and not something the elderly really need?

2. Regulation—"Do we see the elderly as a vulnerable population that needs state oversight?"

— If the door *is* opened to continuing care retirement communities, "we would want to have some regulation."
— New York State's history/philosophy/political climate would require some state oversight of such a program.
— Potential for fraud is there, as the record of past incidents shows.

3. If then continuing care retirement communities were to be permitted, *what* "is it that we want to regulate and who is to regulate it?" Areas that need to be discussed:

— certification and accreditation of operation and program
— financial regulations, disclosure, reserve funds, escrow, and bankruptcy provisions
— involvement of third partner in financing and regulation
— Should there be model provider-resident agreements submitted for state agency approval?
— What about the whole question of Medicaid involvement, eligibility?
— Should resident councils be mandated? How should residents' rights be protected?

4. Issue of advertising and prospectus

— Who or what is to supervise the area of public information when CCRCs are advertised, sold?

— If the focus is on the financial aspects of the program, or the community, then who would supervise: the insurance dept.? the security dept.? the housing dept.? the finance dept.? the banking dept.?

— If the focus is on the service aspects of the communities, then are we talking about supervision from the department of the aging? social services? health? or some new agency?

Given all these questions, perhaps instead of a provider or other organizational body developing a model or demonstration project, the approach should start at the opposite end: ask the state agencies to develop a model regulatory system (before organizations are encouraged to develop programs and apply).

Other issues and concerns discussed by this panel:

— "We do have programs and models in New York State that we can build on. Maybe the most constructive way to go about. . . the development and regulation of these programs is to see what we have out there. . .what it is that we want to create on top of that. . ." Possibly the result would be an option similar to some type of CCRC as now found in other states.

— By involving the state in permitting the development of such communities, "are we in fact encouraging a two-tier service model?" Will the end result be retirement communities for the middle class, and nursing homes for the poorer people who do not have access to the financial resources required for investment in CCRCs? What would be the state's role in preventing this? What would be the state's role in studying/adapting a model so that CCRCs would also be available to people in the lower income brackets?

Suggestions: "Though we didn't come out with firm recommendations and firm conclusions, the sense of both discussion groups, yesterday and today, . . . was

— that New York State public policy should begin to permit the opening of the door for the development of some model of CCRCs;

— that [the State] should . . . probably build on what we already have and see how that can be expanded/extended;

— that if we do have [CCRCs], there is no question that in New York State we would want to have some kind of regulation . . .''

For now, a lot more input is needed from potential consumers about what is really needed. Information from other states is limited; we need to know from our own population.

Finally, we need to "really begin to think through how to regulate, who should regulate, and what should be regulated."[*]

Workshop B. Legal Issues and Barriers

Reporting: James Sanderson,
workshop leader,
partner Tobin and Dempf,
Albany, NY

1. First task of This Panel—Define "Continuing Care"

Definition established: "Continuing Care—independent living with a health care component; not a priority admission into the health care facility but a continuing care agreement providing health care."

And it was noted that given this definition, "nobody is really providing continuing care in New York State."

2. Impediments Involved in Continuing Care

a. Health Dept.—two things here:

— #414.16
— Certificate of Need (CON). Strict process—actually a moratorium now. Also, continuing care could not meet certain other criteria for exemption because it "doesn't . . . take patients from acute care and medicaid patients."

---

[*]In the Q&A that followed this presentation, participants raised further questions, expressed their own views about what the state should do next (relax provisions, seek more information, encourage demonstration projects, avoid a regulatory mess, etc.), and addressed the two-tier health delivery system issue.

b. Department of Social Service regulations
c. The Insurance Law
d. The Attorney General's office
e. The Division of Housing

After discussing all of these "impediments," the workshop participants chose not to take a position, but rather to set forth alternatives and options—some of which, many acknowledged, have "real broad public policy implications."

3. Options

a. Can file an application and see whether it's possible to "tough it out." (But that application will probably "go sideways and get knocked backwards," because of so many of these other impediments."

b. Can try to change the regulations. Agreement with the point made in discussion that the proper first contact is the Governor's office. This issue is so bound up in so many departments, is so tied to the "bureaucratic morass," it's best to have policy come "from above." In fact, assuming that "we go for continuing care in New York," somebody at this conference ought to prepare an application that sets forth a continuing care proposal. This will raise the issues.

c. Can try to "get around" one aspect of the CON issue, but this suggestion has broad public policy implications: needing health beds (if a community is really to provide continuing care) makes the facility subject to CON regulations. But there is a moratorium in New York on health care beds. So—the applicant makes this an exception from the CON, in return promising "never to make the facility eligible for Medicaid." This maneuver would put a facility on an entirely private pay basis—perhaps not a good concept, but one way around a problem.

4. Legislation

There is in existence now a Model Act for Continuing Care, a disclosure act with a limited regulatory oversight position. Mr. Sanderson and Gary Heher of New Jersey were instrumental in preparing this Act which is part of the American Association of Homes for the Aging.

Workshop C. *Financial and Actuarial Aspects*

Recorder: Alwyn Powell, Assistant Professor of Actuarial Science
and Insurance,
Georgia State University;
President/Consulting Actuary of A.V. Powell &
Associates, Inc.,
Philadelphia, Pa.

Recorder Powell reported that Workshop C was divided into two parts: an informative session on how to go about starting a Continuing Care Retirement Community, and a discussion of actuarial concerns.

Major issue discussed: "how do you go about funding the contract?"

a. Should it be funded on a fee-for-service basis, wherein you "bundle the health guarantee" and minimize the risk of the unknown liability of future health care? This alternative restricts the market to a more affluent population which can afford those fees—once transferred to the health care center.

b. Should there be some type of insurance-funding approach—wherein some of the risks are pooled?

Considering some of the informational issues first:

1. Ingredients for Starting a CCRC

a. Site selection
b. Market feasibility study
c. Formation of a project development team. This team, it was felt, should not be a committee in the usual sense of that term. Rather, it should be a team composed of a leader and other necessary professionals: an architect, a marketing consultant, a feasibility consultant, legal counsel, and financial consultant. The Development, or planning, process may last one to two years.
d. Decisions

— Size of community. Relevant statistic here: a minimum of 175 units to be economically feasible
— Type(s) of facilities & accommodations to be offered

— Income level to be targeted
— Contract provisions/Refund provisions
— Type of health care guarantees

e. Financial mechanisms

— Tax free bonds
— Taxable bonds
— Government supported programs
— Conventional mortgages

2. *The Investment Banking Viewpoing Re: Financing the Community*

This was considered a *key* issue in terms of raising the money to get the community off the ground. Basically, there are two types of financing in this regard:

a. A ''substitution effect'' involving a bank loan or credit

b. Credit of the organization—''by far the dominant option''

There are eight issues the investment banking establishment tends to look at:

a. The sponsor, and the sponsor's commitment to the organization

b. Nursing home availability. Controversy here: some feeling a nursing home should be on site, others feeling one should simply be close by and accessible.

c. Competition. If there is another community in the area, how is it doing?

d. Market penetration. Who can afford the community? What percentage of the target population is needed?

e. Financial feasibility. Type of reserves needed. Experience/ expertise of consultant.

f. Pre-sales. Often 50% pre-sales is used as a guideline, this being achieved even before construction or opening. It is better to stop development and take losses prior to major bond issues—if pre-sales are inadequate.

g. Professional management. *Who* will administer the community?

h. Type of services, contract guarantee, and pricing of same.

3. Actuarial Issues

a. Continuing care appears to be a cost efficient delivery system from a utilization perspective for providing long-term care to the elderly.

b. The "traditional" continuing care concept, where fees do not vary according to the living status (apartment versus nursing care) of the resident, is affordable by a much larger percentage than is currently being served by the industry; this percentage is probably not less than 10% and may be as large as 25% or more of the elderly population.

c. The "middle to upper income" designation is probably correct for what is referred to as "the traditional continuing care contract"—one where the resident does not pay an additional fee when transferring to the health care center. Question here: how do you fund this health care transfer? One approach: "unbundle it." Have a fee for service system. Advantage here is minimizing risk of underestimating future health care cost. Disadvantage: restricts your potential market.

d. Residents may run out of money once they are in the community; as a rule, they are not asked to leave unless they have "willfully dissipate[d]" their monies. This is a concern of the policy makers when deciding whether or not to "let CCRCs enter."

e. If some type of insurance funding is undertaken, very careful planning is required. Many of the communities that have experienced problems with the continuing care contract simply did not have proper tools or information available for prudent planning re: funding their health care obligation. In other words, the problem lies not with the concept of continuing care, but with inadequate information and planning.

4. Some Final Thoughts Re: "Potential Regulation and What Should Be Considered Here"

a. The actuarial data base for CCRCs is very thin. Data needs to be collected, and a regulatory authority may wish to require this. And funds should be provided so that this data can be analyzed on a regular basis to develop standard tables.

b. "How do you define insolvency?" Need to consider how cash flow relates to insurance funding, to actuarial solvency.

c. What are the objectives of regulation?

— Consumer protection
— Early warning system
— Standardization of benefits
— Model contracts/refunds

d. Is the cost of imposing some type of detailed actuarial regulation really worth the benefits of preventing future losses?

In the course of the discussion that followed, Recorder Alwyn Powell clarified an earlier statement: there are two approaches to funding the continuing care concept. One is the unbundled approach. And one is an insurance approach. Both have their advantages and disadvantages, and the point was that the regulatory authority should review same.

The unbundled approach poses less risk to the community, but more risk to the individual. With the insurance approach, it is the reverse.

Workshop D. *Programmatic and Operational Problems*

Recorder: Daniel Sambol,
                 Director,
                 Division on Aging,
                 Protestant Welfare Agencies, Inc.,
                 New York City

Since New York State does not permit CCRCs, this session was fortunate to have among its participants persons from Massachusetts, New Jersey and Pennsylvania with direct experience in establishing and operating CCRCs.

1. A Review of Apparent Differences Between Current Approaches Utilized by the Nonprofit Sector in New York State in Existing, Long-Term Care Service Systems, and Those of the Proposed CCRCs

a. In New York, the nonprofit sector is geared to serving dependent and needy populations. CCRCs, by comparison, serve a more affluent population with high levels of service expectations.

b. In New York, the long-term care system is health-oriented and geared to institutional services. By comparison, CCRCs focus on a residential model, accommodations for independent, ambulatory, "well-elderly" with health care services available but not emphasized. This is even reflected in the architectural design of the communities.

c. The nonprofit's corporate structure would have to be reconsidered with respect to its not-for-profit status, "the possibility of receiving unrelated business income and its status as Medicare-Medicaid provider."

d. Admissions policies. In a CCRC, the service package must be sold, and a written contract must spell out the responsibilities and obligations of both parties.

2. Certificate of Need

This is an important factor in attempting to move ahead with CCRCs in New York State. Since CCRCs combine housing and health services, it is unlikely that Certificate-of-Need approval could be obtained in today's climate.

3. Overlooked Factor

New York State officials consider the State progressive, relative to monies spent on institutional care. But they overlook the value of appropriate housing (CCRCs?) in keeping people *out of* skilled nursing facilities. "Since the CCRC does not stress health but focuses on a secure residence with many support services, its important preventive elements may be overlooked in New York State."

4. Comment

It was suggested that New York State, the only state to prohibit CCRCs, might be benefitting from this prohibition in terms of gaining time to learn from other states' experiences. Question: is subsidy needed for CCRCs? If so, how can such subsidy be arranged? Would the housing unit have to subsidize the health facility? Comment from a developer in another state: operational issues must be examined before opening any community. The question must be asked: is there a market for such a community? In New York, subsidized housing (Section 202, Section 8) has inevitable waiting lists, whereas CCRCs require promotion—marketing is the key.

5. Other Commentary

a. CCRCs must be *sold*. Persons do not buy unless informed of services and value. Emphasis must be placed on independent living units

— social, recreational and dining facilities
— luxurious and gracious lifestyle
— health care services that are available when needed
— the "non-institutional" nature of the program
— available health care services: a skilled nursing facility, outpatient clinic, home health and home care services.

b. The CCRC financial package requires an up-front investment by the resident, plus a monthly maintenance fee. The contract spells out services and fees, and permits residents to budget accordingly. The contract is not a real estate contract, but New York State treats it as if it were, requiring a prospectus that must include a listing of all possible risks.

c. CCRCs serve independent people intent on preserving a certain type of lifestyle. Quality of food, maintenance and housekeeping are major issues. Resident associations are vehicles for articulate demands.

d. While sizes of CCRCs vary, they are rarely developed with less than 200 units plus 60 skilled nursing facility beds.

Questions raised in discussion involved

— rental to outsiders,
— having young people around,
— quality of service being critical to the success of a CCRC,
— financial feasibility as a delicate area,
— feasibility studies: *essential* items, but who should do?
— permitting the CCRC's skilled nursing facility to be open to the public at first, with CCRC residents becoming priority patients,
— attracting the applicant in his sixties, when the average population has aged "in place" to 82, and
— the necessity of pre-sales.

Conclusion

There seemed to be a consensus that CCRCs offered valuable services to a significant sector of the elderly population and should be explored. It was proposed that follow-up conferences be held periodically so that those planning the development of CCRCs could share their experiences, successes and frustrations in order to help one another move ahead.

Workshop E. Consumer Interests

Reporting: Marcia Steinhauer, Ph.D.,
Associate Professor,
Graduate Program of Administration,
Rider College,
Lawrenceville, NJ

The State of New York is at a critical stage in the matter of support for Continuing Care Retirement Communities. As noted earlier in this conference, ". . . in times of crisis, one is given to exaggeration . . ." and perhaps we are now witnessing exaggeration in regard to the CCRC.

The clearest arguments in support of the CCRC either in or out of this state appear to be two documented observations: (1) the new census data shows that three years have been added to the American life span within a single decade; and (2) there are multiple disabilities associated with increased age.

The combination of these phenomena requires a residential setting that provides for complete independence and a full range of services. Moreover, these services should be calibrated to the changing needs of the individual.

There seems to be every reason to include the CCRC among the range of innovative ways of coping with the dual desires of older persons for both independence and security. The participants of this workshop would also encourage housing and health care professionals to pursue creative alternatives rather than strictly institutional placements.

Because of these reasons and the fact that the State of New York is losing valuable human and financial resources, the Consumer Interests Workshop offers the following suggestions:

1. There should be an opportunity within the State of New York to develop the CCRC concept.
2. Public and consumer education should include explanations of the concept of CCRC as being not just a nursing home and should emphasize to older individuals the importance of entering a CCRC while they are still active.
3. The Consumer Protection Board should be a focal point within the state for protecting the future of the elderly. This board should have early involvement in the development of CCRCs.
4. There should be legislation to assure the financial resources of CCRCs to secure against their non-failure.
5. CCRCs should include the potential utilization of insurance policies as part of the entrance fees to stabilize financial feasibility.
6. It should be recognized that the health care component is but one aspect of the total CCRC concept. This notion should be put in the proper perspective by the health bureaucracy in its oversight activities of CCRCs.
7. The development of CCRCs should be encouraged to make them economically feasible for the aging population.

EPILOGUE

The Conference Planning Committee wishes to emphasize that the proceedings of the recent conference, summarized in the preceding pages, simply illuminate—not resolve—a complex subject. This is in keeping with the intent of the Conference.

The subject—the future of continuing care retirement communities in New York State—remains short of simple solution. short even of unanimous opinion about the advisability of encouraging, through legal provision, the establishment of life care communities in New York. It is clear, however, that while the State of New York acted early to protect the assets and well-being of elderly in need of long-term care, it has done little to encourage upper-middle-class citizens to remain within the State in their later years.

New York's attention to, and investment in, the well-being of its poor and moderate-income elderly citizens is highly commendable and establishes fine models for other states. However, the State's lack of attention to its self-supporting retirees (usually in the middle and upper-middle income brackets), and its failure to encourage these citizens to remain in the State in resident modes of their choice, have created an exodus to other states where life care or continuing care communities abound. Thus, New York State loses many retired citizens whose vitality, initiative and capital investments in their earning years contributed greatly to the State's strength. In fact, New York loses their *continued* economic contributions.

Organizations—nonprofit and proprietary both—wishing to address the housing and health care needs of independent retirees come up against inhibiting factors in New York. The lack of clarity in law and regulation concerning continuing care retirement communities makes necessary testing in the courts, an expensive process which inhibits even the most fearless, potential sponsor/developer. The number of governmental departments having overlapping jurisdiction in the creation of communities desiring to add long-term care and on-going health care provisions discourages even those experienced in dealing with government. Overall, the lack of government encouragement to those interested in establishing continuing care retirement communities actually inhibits the creation of such communities.

These indirect but nevertheless prohibitive inhibitions appear to do a disservice to those elderly who, with their own assets, would prefer to live in retirement communities in New York such as have been successful in the neighboring states of New Jersey, Connecticut, Pennsylvania, Massachusetts and many other localities. Such self-supporting retirees wish to reside near remaining family and friends in security and contentment, knowing that if infirmity makes it impossible to continue a self-sustaining lifestyle, prior agreements guarantee proper care with dignity.

If the Conference has begun a process of illumination for framers of public policy it will have achieved its purpose.

Suggested Readings

Adelmann, N. *Directory of life care communities.* 2nd edition, Kennett Square: Kendal Crosslands, 1980.

Berry, R. and Weaver, B. *Life table estimation and financial evaluation for California life care homes.* Berkeley: Teknekron Research, Inc., 1980.

Cohen, D.L. Continuing-care communities for the elderly: Potential pitfalls and proposed legislation. *University of Pennsylvania Law Review,* 1980, *128-849,* 883-936.

Consumers Guide to Independent Living for Older Americans, published by Life Care Society of America Inc., Doylestown, Pa., 1980.

Continuing Care Homes: A Guidebook for Consumers, published by the American Association of Homes for the Aging, Washington, D.C., 1976.

Dilgard, C.K. *Financial management guide for nonprofit homes for the aging.* Evanston: Health and Welfare Ministries Division, Board of Global Ministries of the United Methodist Church, 1978.

Greene, M.R. Life care centers—a new concept in insurance. *Journal of Risk and Insurance,* 1981, *48,* 403-421.

Hewitt, D.L. Actuarial amortization of entry fees for life care communities. *1981-82 Proceedings of the Conference of Actuaries in Public Practice,* 1982, *31,* 506-523.

Parr, J. and Green, S. *Housing environments of elderly persons: Typology and discriminant analysis.* Clearwater, FL: Foundation for Aging Research, 1981.

Rose, A.M. *Lifecare industry 1982.* Philadelphia: Laventhol and Horwath, 1981.

Sosnoff, H.D. and Blumenthal, J.E. Accommodation fees: Have you earned them? *American Health Care Journal,* 1980, Jan. 6(1) 23-25.

Steinhauer, M.B. and Ecker, J.S. Life care communities: Private sector involvement in housing alternatives for the elderly. Paper presented at the annual meeting of the Gerontological Society of America, San Diego, November, 1980.

Trueblood-Raper, A. (Ed.) *National Continuing Care Directory* for AAHA American Association of Homes for the Aging, published by AARP American Association of Retired Persons, Washington, D.C.; Scott Foresman & Company, Lifelong Learning Division, Glenview, Ill., 1984.

Turner, L., Schreter, C., Zetick, B., Weisbrod, G., Pollakowski, H., *Housing options for the community resident elderly: Policy report of the housing choices of the older american study.* Graduate School of Social Work and Social Research: Bryn Mawr College, 1982.

Wasser, L.J. and Cloud, D.A. (eds.) *Continuing care: Issues for nonprofit providers,* Washington, D.C.: American Association of Homes for the Aging, 1978.

Winklevoss, H.E. and Powell, A.V. *Continuing care retirement communities: An empirical, financial, and legal analysis.* Published for: The Pension Research Council of the Wharton School, University of Pennsylvania, by Richard D. Irwin, Inc., Homewood, Ill., 1984.

Winklevoss, H.E. and Powell, A.V. *1982 reference directory of continuing care retirement communities.* Philadelphia: Human Services Research, Inc., 1982.

Winklevoss, H.E. and Powell, A.V. Retirement communities: Assessing the liability of alternative health care guarantees. *Journal of Long-Term Care Administration.* 1981, *9,* 8-33.

Conference Speakers and Panelists

David Adest
Partner
Loeb & Troper
Certified Public Accountants
270 Madison Avenue
New York, N.Y. 10016

Ruth Bennett, Ph.D.
Deputy Director
Center for Geriatrics and
    Gerontology
Columbia University
100 Haven Ave.
New York, N.Y. 10032

David L. Cohen, Esq.
Associate
Ballard, Spahr, Andrews and
    Ingersoll
30 South 17th Street
Philadelphia, Pa. 19103

Patricia Cook
Member of the Board
Loretto Geriatric Center
3628 Pheasant Lane
Endwell, N.Y. 13760

John J. Costello
Byrne, Costello & Pickard
Attorneys at Law
499 Warren Building
Syracuse, N.Y. 13202

Craig A. Duncan
Executive Director
James A. Eddy Memorial
    Geriatric Center
2224 Burdett Avenue
Troy, N.Y. 12180

Frank E. Elliott
Chairman of the Board
Life Care Society of America,
    Inc.
Ferry and Lion Hill Roads
Doylestown, Pa. 18901

Monsignor Charles Fahey
Director
Third Age Center
Fordham University
New York, N.Y. 10023

Barry J. Gurland, M.D.
Director
Center for Geriatrics and
    Gerontology
Columbia University
100 Haven Ave.
New York, N.Y. 10032

Garrett M. Heher, Esq.
Smith, Stratton, Wise, Heher
    & Brennan
One Palmer Square
Princeton, N.J. 08540

Melvin Katz
Manager
Caring for the Aging Practice
Peat, Marwick, Mitchell & Co.
345 Park Avenue
New York, N.Y. 10154

Laurence F. Lane
Director for Non-Profit and
    Special Programs
American Health Care
    Association
1200 15th Street NW
Washington, D.C. 20005

Abraham Monk, Ph.D.
Director
Brookdale Institute on Aging
 and Adult Human
 Development
Columbia University
422 West 113th Street
New York, N.Y. 10027

Ian Morrison, Ed.D.
President
Greer-Woodycrest
R.R.2, Box 1000
Millbrook, N.Y. 12545

Lloyd Nurick
Director
New York Association of
 Homes and Services for the
 Aging
194 Washington Ave.
Albany, N.Y. 12210

Corinne Plummer
Deputy Commissioner
Division of Adult Services
New York State Department
 of Social Services
40 North Pearl Street
Albany, N.Y. 12243

Alwyn V. Powell
President
A.V. Powell & Associates,
 Inc.
40 Marietta Street, NW
Suite 1320
Atlanta, Ga. 30303-2812

Aaron M. Rose, C.P.A.
Laventhol & Horwath
Certified Public Accountants
1845 Walnut Street
Philadelphia, Pa. 19103

Daniel Sambol
Director
Division on Aging
Federation of Protestant
 Welfare Agencies, Inc.
281 Park Avenue South
New York, N.Y. 10010

James W. Sanderson, Esq.
Tobin & Dempf
100 State Street
Albany, N.Y. 12207

Doris Schwartz, FAAN
Resident
Foulkeways L-110
Gwynedd, Pa. 19436

William B. Sims
President
Herbert J. Sims & Co., Inc.
77 Water Street
New York, N.Y.

Marcia B. Steinhauer, Ph.D.
Associate Professor
Graduate Program for
 Administrators
Rider College
Lawrenceville, N.J. 08648

Erika Teutsch
Metropolitan Area Coordinator
 for Adult Services
New York State Department
 for Social Services
2 World Trade Center
New York, N.Y. 10047

George Warner, M.D.
Special Health Care Advisor
Health Facilities Standards
  and Control
State of New York Department
  of Health
Office of Health Systems
  Management
Tower Building
Empire State Plaza
Albany, N.Y. 12237

Howard E. Winklevoss, Ph.D.
President
Winklevoss & Associates
3700 Science Center
Philadelphia, Pa. 19104

David E. Wilder, Ph.D.
Deputy Director
Center for Geriatrics and
  Gerontology
Columbia University
100 Haven Ave.
New York, N.Y. 10032

Conference Participants

Leo E. Baldwin
Senior Coordinator, Housing
AARP
1909 K Street, N.W.
Washington, DC 20049

Rose Boritzer
Administrator
Kingsbridge Heights Nursing
    Home
3400 Cannon Place
Bronx, NY 10463

Robert Borsody, Esq.
250 Park Avenue, 14th Floor
New York, NY 10177

Martin L. Brothers, Esq.
Attorney at Law
250 West 57th Street
New York, NY 10019

Sylva Brunner
Executive Director
Swiss Benevolent Society of
    New York
37 West 67th Street
New York, NY 10023

Marlene Burnett
Planning Associate
Church Charity Foundation
    of L.I.
393 Front Street
Hempstead, NY 11550

James W. Butler, Jr.
Ernest and Whinney
14th Floor, Commerce Tower
1 Commerce Square
Memphis, Tennessee 38103

Dr. Vivian Carlin
Supervisor
Planning and Policy Analysis
New Jersey State Division
    on Aging
CN 807
Trenton, NJ 08625

Carlos Castro
Controller
Amsterdam House
1060 Amsterdam Avenue
New York, NY 10025

Ken Chernoff
Administrator
Medical Center for Aging
Doylestown, Pa. 18901

Reverend William Coleman
San Simeon by the Sound
Box W
Greenport, NY 11944

Beth Collins
Senior Program Specialist
Division of Adult Services
NYS Department of Social
    Services
40 North Pearl Street
Albany, NY 12243

David Conover, Architect
Conover/Elton Associates
P.O. Box 492
Boston, Mass. 02123

Kathleen Cook
Director of Research and
    Planning
General Health Management,
    Inc.
3 Barnard Lane
Bloomfield, Ct. 06002

Phillip Cotterill
Acting Director
Division of Economic Analysis
Office of Research
Health Care Financing
    Administration
330 Independence Avenue,
    S.W.
Washington, DC 20201

Sarah Craig
Assistant Deputy Administrator
Long Term Care
Medical Assistance Program
330 West 34th Street
New York, NY 10001

Bob Daino
Vice President
Continental Securities
    Corporation
P.O. Box 2308
Syracuse, NY 13220

Robert Dermody
L. Dermody, Burk and Brown
Powelson Building
Syracuse, NY 13202

Reverend Leonard DiFalco
St. Ann's Parish
854 Midland Avenue
Yonkers, NY 10704

Vincent DiRubbio
Administrator
St. John's Episcopal Home
    for Aged and Blind
452 Herkimer Street
Brooklyn, NY 11213

Helen T. Dodd
Board Member
Orange County Home for
    Aged Women
27 South Street
Middletown, NY 10940

Anne Dowling
Deputy Commissioner
NYS Division of Housing and
    Community Renewal
2 World Trade Center
New York, NY 10047

Patricia Farrell
36 Bobolink Road
Yonkers, NY 10701

Susan T. Farwell
Consultant
Peat, Marwick, Mitchell & Co.
345 Park Avenue
New York, NY 10154

Thomas Ford, Esq.
Hahn, Hahn & Ford
105 Hillside Avenue
Williston Park, NY 11596

Jerry Frishberg
President
Life Care Communities
   Corporation
2 Bala Plaza, Suite 714
Bala Cynwyd, Pa. 19004

Neil L. Gaynes
Neil L. Gaynes and Associates,
   Inc.
481 Ridge Road
Highland Park, Ill. 60035

Joan Gibson
Regional Aging Program
   Specialist
AoA Region II/OHD/DHHS
26 Federal Plaza, Room 4149
New York, NY 10278

Linda Gowdy
Assistant to Senator Tarky
   Lombardi, Jr.
The Senate
State of New York
Albany, NY 12247

John H. Gunder
Director
Information Systems
Life Care Society of America
Doylestown, Pa. 18901

Lawrence Hall
Continental Securities
   Corporation
P.O. Box 2308
Syracuse, NY 13220

Ralph E. Hall
Senior Vice President
Morningside House Nursing
   Home
1000 Pelham Parkway
Bronx, NY 10461

Norman E. Harper
President
Loretto Geriatric Center
700 East Brighton Avenue
Syracuse, New York 13205

Ray Hartmann
Assistant Administrator
Eger Lutheran Home
140 Meisner Avenue
Staten Island, NY 10306

Marsel Heisel
Director of Curriculum
Institute on Aging
Rutgers University
43 Mine Street
New Brunswick, NJ 08903

David Hodgkins
Director
Bureau of Residential Health
   Care Facilities
NYS Department of Health
Albany, NY 12237

Charlotte Holstein, Chairperson
Board of Directors
Loretto Geriatric Center
700 East Brighton Avenue
Syracuse, NY 13205

George R. Hughes, Esq.
Associate
Semmes, Bowen & Semmes
10 Light Street
Baltimore, Md. 21202

Maresa Isaacs
The Alpha Center
73-16 Wisconsin Avenue,
   Suite 400
Bethesda, Md. 20814

David Jepson
Jeter, Cook and Jepson
799 Main Street
Hartford, Connecticut 06103

Saul S. Katz
Associate Attorney
New York State Division of
    Housing and Community
    Renewal
2 World Trade Center
New York, NY 10047

Gerald Katzman, Esq.
22 First Street
Troy, NY 12180

Barbara Kleger
Director of Development
Life Care Communities
    Corporation
2 Bala Plaza, Suite 714
Bala Cynwyd, Pa. 19004

Reverend Donald Kraft
The Wartburg Home
Bradley Avenue
Mount Vernon, NY 10552

Kenneth Kuhnle
Controller
Life Care Society of America
Pine Run Community
Doylestown, Pa. 18901

Nelson Leenhouts, President
Home Leasing Corporation
371 White Spruce Blvd.
Rochester, NY 14623

Faustina Lees
North Shore Unitarian Society
12 Jeanette Drive
Port Washington, NY 11050

Robert Leibenluft, Esq.
Hogan & Hartson
815 Connecticut Avenue
Washington, DC 20006

Reverend Phillip Lewis
Vice President, Pastoral Care
Church Charity Foundation of
    Long Island
36 Cathedral Avenue
Garden City, NY 11530

Eleanor Little
Administrator
Good Shepherd-Fairview Home
80 Fairview Avenue
Binghamton, NY 13904

Mary Lucier
Special Assistant
Life Care Society of America
Doylestown, Pa. 18901

Jane M. Lyons
Associate Executive Director
Sea View Home and Hospital
460 Brielle Avenue
Staten Island, NY 10314

Michael McGarvey, M.D.
Chief Medical Liaison
Department of Psychiatry
St. Vincent's Hospital and
    Medical Center of New
    York
7th Avenue and 11th Street
New York, NY 10011

Frank Mandy
Policy Analyst
NY Association of Homes for
    the Aging
194 Washington Avenue
Albany, NY 12210

Harold Margolin
Vice President and Manager
Supportive Living Projects Unit
Merrill Lynch
White Weld Capital
 Markets Group
One Liberty Plaza
165 Broadway
New York, NY 10080

Luba P. Mebert,
Executive Director
House of Holy Comforter
2751 Grand Concourse
Bronx, NY 10468

Harold C. Mufson
Administrator
Swiss Home of Mount Kisco
53 Mountain Avenue
Mount Kisco, NY 10549

Edward Munns
Munns and Dobbins
700 White Plains Road
Scarsdale, NY 10583

Thomas N. Pappas
Vice President
Winklevoss & Associates
3700 Science Center
Philadelphia, Pa. 19104

Barbara Parkoff
New Jersey Division on Aging
CN 807
Trenton, NJ 08625

Linda Paton
Foulkeways S-4
Gwynedd, Pa. 19436

Harvey E. Pies
Gardner, Carton & Douglas
1875 Bye Street, NW
Washington, DC 20006

Rachel Pohl
Research Assistant
Public Policy and
 Administration
435 West 119th Street, 6-F
New York, NY 10027

Thomas Powers
Vice President
Goodkin Research
275 Commercial Boulevard
Lauderdale by the Sea, Fla.
 33308

Michael Pulling
Health Care Management
 Associates
194 Washington Avenue
4th Floor
Albany, NY 12210

Ann Trueblood Raper
Consultant in Gerontology
6002 34th Place, N.W.
Washington, DC 20015

Amey Rulon-Miller
Policy Specialist
American Association of
 Homes for the Aging
1050 Seventeenth Street,
 N.W., Suite 700
Washington, DC 20036

John P. Ryan
Assistant Administrator
Frances Schervier Home and
 Hospital
2975 Independence Avenue
Bronx, NY 10463

Al Schwartz
Federation of Jewish
 Philanthropies
130 East 59th Street
New York, NY 10022

Henry D. Sedgwick, President
Retirement Centers Group, Inc.
126 West 80th Street
New York, NY 10024

Abraham Seiman
Associate Director
Wartburg Lutheran Home for
the Aging
2598 Fulton Street
Brooklyn, NY 11207

Pamela Shea
OKM Associates
148 State Street
Boston, Massachusetts 02109

Marilyn Shilkoff, Ed.D.
Consultant
25 Larchmont Avenue
Larchmont, NY 10538

Eleanor Snow
Member, Board of Managers
Orange County Home for Aged
Women
27 South Street
Middletown, NY 10940

Carl Spencer
Director
Syracuse Research Corporation
Merrill Lane
Syracuse, NY 13210

Mary E. Sughrue
Special Assistant
Medicaid Fraud Control
270 Broadway, 17th Floor
New York, NY 10007

Allan Thomas
Coordinator for Gerontology
Services
St. Francis Hospital
North Road
Poughkeepsie, NY 12601

Paul A. Wagner
President
NPO/TASK FORCE, Inc.
124 East 40th Street
New York, NY 10016

Mitchell Waife
Administrator
Jewish Home and Hospital for
the Aged
120 West 106th Street
New York, NY 10025

James B. Weil
Vice President
Metropolitan Life Insurance
Co.
1 Madison Avenue
New York, NY 10010

Gary Whitworth
President
Adventist Living Centers
15 Salt Creek Lane
Hinsdale, Illinois 60521

Stephen F. Wiggins
General Atlantic
120 East 55th Street
New York, NY 10022